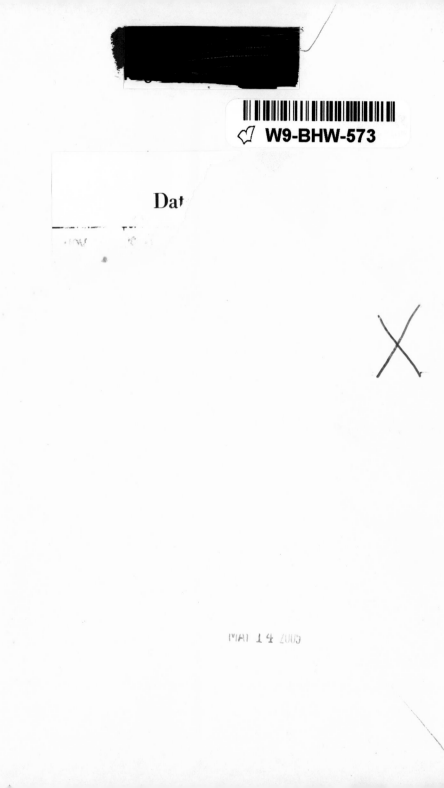

Dat

Healing
Our
Health Care
System

Healing
Our
Health Care
System

♦

LEONARD ABRAMSON

GROVE WEIDENFELD

New York

Published by Grove Weidenfeld
A division of Wheatland Corporation
841 Broadway
New York, NY 10003-4793

Published in Canada by General Publishing Company, Ltd.

Library of Congress Cataloging-in-Publication Data
Abramson, Leonard.
Healing our health care system / Leonard Abramson. — 1st ed.
p.   cm.
1. Medical care—United States.   2. Medical economics—United
States.   I. Title.
[DNLM: 1. Delivery of Health Care—United States.   2. Health
Services—United States.   W 84 AA1 A15h]
RA395.A3A477   1990
362.1'0973—dc20
DNLM/DLC
for Library of Congress   89-71515
                                                                              CIP

ISBN 0-8021-1257-9

Manufactured in the United States of America

Printed on acid-free paper

Designed by Jill Weber

First Edition 1990

1   3   5   7   9   10   8   6   4   2

THIS BOOK IS DEDICATED TO
THE FIRST TRUE BELIEVER,
MY WIFE, MADLYN

ACKNOWLEDGMENTS

I wish to thank many talented, concerned people for their help in my writing of this book, including Michael F. Avellone, D.O., John H. Glick, M.D., Robert L. Goodman, M.D., Hyman R. Kahn, M.D., Arthur N. Leibowitz, M.D., Jay R. Rosan, D.O., Neil Schlackman, M.D., David B. Soll, M.D., Michael A. Stocker, M.D., Robert J. Wolfson, M.D., who all shared with me many insights from their years of medical practice.

Alan R. Letofsky, Esq., for helping with the complex medical-legal aspects of the book.

Marshall Rozzi and James Broderick, who gave me the benefit of their years in the hospital industry.

Melvin Stein, for his work in developing a program for large companies to use when selecting and evaluating health insurance.

Isadore Barmash, who helped to direct and discipline my writing and to make it more readable.

To Esther Eavenson, my secretary, a very special thanks for working long hours deciphering my dictation and interpreting my handwriting, and then typing the many drafts of the manuscript.

Finally, love and gratitude to my three daughters, Marcy, Nancy, and Judith, who have always been the most important part of my life and were the true reasons behind my striving for excellence.

C O N T E N T S

INTRODUCTION

This book was written for all Americans. It did not start out that way. My original concept was to write a book solely for the senior executives who lead America's organizations. I was not trying to be elitist; I was endeavoring to reach the people with the most clout to help reform the American health care system. I wanted to address the decision-makers to help them understand our health care delivery system, to share with them the knowledge needed to make positive changes in the planning, financing, and delivery of, and accountability for, the medical care of their employees, their families, and fellow Americans.

Sometime during the outlining and drafting process, it became apparent to me that I was writing for a broader audience. I was not just writing about a multibillion-dollar industry but about our health and the quality of all of our lives. If the telephone calls and letters that I receive daily mean anything, many of you are interested, and you would like to do something about a system you know needs help. You want information and a plan of action, and I will try to provide both.

In the chapters that follow, I will share much of what I have learned in twenty-five years in health care. It will then be up to you to act. If you are the president of a company, this book will show you how to evaluate and improve the health care benefits provided to your employees and how to save money. If you are an individual, this book will show how to evaluate and improve the health care you and your family receive and how to save money.

This book will also discuss some of the debates taking place in the continuing drama that I call the psychoneuroeconomics of American medicine. You will learn about funding mechanisms and the roles played by the federal government, insurance companies, industry, unions, and others. I will give you an inside look at the operations of hospitals, physicians, clinical laboratories, pharmaceutical companies, insurance companies, health maintenance organizations (HMOs), self-insured plans, trust funds, and jointly funded programs and their interactions with unions and employers. We will discuss these and other mechanisms to help you understand their place in the evolution of our health care system and the place they may have in the future.

Reading this book will give you the inside information to master a methodology. You will also be able to write your own report cards for various health care delivery systems and analytically question and hold accountable various health care delivery components to which you are exposed. My goal is to try to help you become informed, knowledgeable, and a probing purchaser of health care whether you are an executive making the purchase for your company or an individual concerned about yourself and your family. In either case, I aim to leave you with some easy ways to analyze and help make decisions about which health care is best for you and those who matter to you. You must take responsible action, so that together we can become an effective force in reshaping the American medical delivery system to more closely meet our country's needs. To do this, Americans and American industry need to take an active role in holding those of us in the health care community accountable, and those of us in the health care community must hold ourselves accountable. All of us must participate. It cannot be left to the individual or to hospitals, physicians, insurance companies, HMOs, or large industry. Plato once said, "No physician insofar as he is a physician, considers his own good in what he prescribes for the good of his patients; the true physician is also a ruler and has the human body as a subject." We must all play an active role in making decisions that result in new policy and a new model for American medical care. I will tell you how and participate myself, but you must get involved if we are to have a medical community that meets the Platonic ideal.

As the founder and chief executive of one of the nation's most successful health maintenance organization companies, I have been fortunate enough to prosper because I understand the health care industry. By applying American capitalism to health care, I have realized the American dream. I see this book as an opportunity for a partial payback. I am anxious to share my knowledge with you so that, together, we may help our country regain its rightful world leadership position in management, industry, economics, and medicine.

Royalties from this book will be contributed to cancer research and treatment.

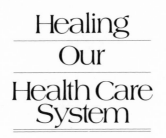

Healing
Our
Health Care
System

CHAPTER ONE

American Health Care: The Staggering Elephant

While a prematurely born infant emits a plaintive wail in the neonatal intensive care unit, a forty-year-old man struggles for life in a respirator, his system still in shock from a massive heart attack. On a lower floor in a quarantine wing, AIDS patients try to bolster one another's spirits. In the geriatric ward, some elderly patients are thankful for their moderate ills, but others wilt under Alzheimer's disease.

The staff moves briskly about in the pragmatic hum of the vast medical center. On the surface, all seems under control. But a head nurse warily eyes her juniors, knowing that a recent, unsettled strike has left a core of unrest among them. At doctors' meetings, physicians casually exchange case experiences, though they, too, are troubled by the increase in cancer patients and by certain infections that appear to be resistant to normally effective drugs. The medical staff is all too aware of AIDS and its rampant infectiousness. And the head of the institution looks ahead unhappily to an imminent meeting with department heads in which runaway budgets will top the agenda and, doubtless, again create hot debate.

All of them, those in the beds and those in the white uniforms, share one thing. They are involved in an American health care system which, while envied by many other countries, bears just beneath the surface such deep scars as spiraling costs, poor cost-effectiveness, inefficient, erratic quality, and misguided marketing efforts. Outside the wards and private rooms are millions of other Americans, many of them covered by health plans and paying more for it every year, but millions of others at or near poverty level remain largely uncovered by any health insurance and are ignored by the health care system.

The numbers are awesome.

With outlays of $600 billion, looming inflation, extreme pressure on profit margins, a rising bite of 12 percent of the gross national product leaping to 15 percent in just a few years—yet with 37 million Americans without health insurance—today's American health megaplex is not a viable entity. Costs are being fueled by rising technology costs, an aging population and a proliferating horde of retirees, providers' excess capacity, and exploding demand. The average American is paying $2,000 a year for health protection. Current employee and retiree costs place an immense burden on both the private and public sectors. These costs already exceed corporate profits in a growing number of cases and could easily bankrupt major corporations in future years.

Authoritative estimates say that about 20 percent of our health care outlays is being wasted, which would mean a total of $120 billion in 1989—a vast sum indeed to be allowed to go down the drain.

How did our health care system get sick? What can be done about it? Or is it just a case of a colossus so unwieldy and unbridled that it would be best left to blunder on?

Not at all. I think that much can be done to help and control the system, make it more efficient and cost-effective. But, first, how did a vital public service such as the nation's health care turn into a swollen, stumbling organism? I suspect that at least a partial answer lies in the fact that a loan is only the beginning of a helping

1. National Health Expenditures

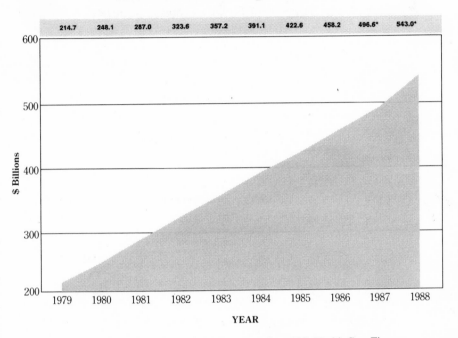

Source: Chart prepared by U.S. Healthcare. Data from U.S. Health Care Financing Administration, *Health Care Financing Review,* summer 1987.

* Estimated.

process. Take the health maintenance organization, the HMO, with federal aid from which our company as well as many others benefited. U.S. Healthcare, Inc., is an innovative company competing in a capitalistic system, generating profits by introducing efficacy and effectiveness into the presently oligarchical health care delivery system. Its competition is conventional health insurance and the provider community content with the status quo. Grants and loans in the form of venture capital were generated by

2. National Health Expenditures
as Percent of Gross National Product

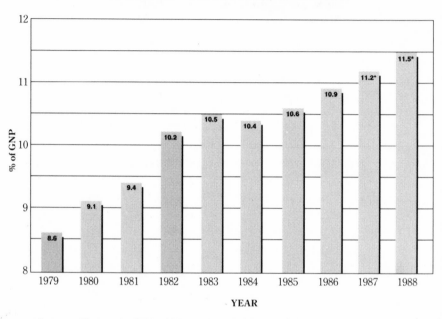

Source: Chart prepared by U.S. Healthcare. Data from U.S. Health Care Financing Administration, *Health Care Financing Review,* summer 1987.

* Estimated.

Public Law 93–222, the HMO Law, which provides much of the impetus for the research and development that fostered the HMO. But the federal government and the HMOs did not mesh or communicate very well after that.

Their attitudes remind one of the centipede and the owl. A centipede with arthritis in its many ankles was making its way through the woods, racked with pain. He looked up and saw a wise old owl in a tree. "Wise old owl," the centipede asked, "how can I cure this painful affliction that I have?" The wise old owl looked down and said, "Well, I can give you a ninety-six percent cure rate." "That's wonderful," the centipede said, "but how can you do that?" The owl replied, "Well, you simply turn yourself into a horse with only four ankles instead of a hundred." As the centipede proceeded down the path, it looked back and said, "But wise old owl, how can a centipede turn itself into a horse?" Said the owl, "Well, I only make policy. It's up to you to implement it."

The wide-open loans and the easy tax-free-bond mechanism and the confusion about how to use them are only a few of the problems that led to an uncontrolled, inefficient health care system. Here are a few other reasons: Finally awakening to the possibilities of twentieth-century marketing, hospitals today are courting doctors on prime-time television, forgetting that their real customers are patients. Hospital administrators, trained to build mammoth institutions, opt for scale, not efficiency. Physicians, most of them honest, sincere practitioners, nonetheless watch silently as others overcharge the system, behaving as if they were businessmen, and refer patients to expensive specialists. In the main tent, the surgery, inefficient practitioners are not rooted out until they commit some form of malpractice. Furthermore, the protective "club" atmosphere created by many doctors can lead to tragic circumstances for patients.

All those factors and others, including the unrealistic estimates of employee costs made by American business, created a crisis situation. The fact is that, with the exception of the federal deficit and the trade imbalance, the nation's health care system is America's biggest domestic problem. As it is set up today, it is also one of our biggest boondoggles. And what is particularly sad is that the numerous solutions at hand are being spurned by many professional practitioners. Americans spend more of their income on health care than any other nationality, but their average life span, infant mortality rate, and death rate do not set the world's standards. Despite our great wealth and our manufacturing, service, and creative capabilities, our health care system is only average among the big industrial nations. And the cost-effectiveness of this vast expenditure is dramatically lacking when measured against performance. Hospitals now suffer greater overcapacity than heavy industry. In 1970 the occupancy rate for U.S. hospitals was 80 percent. In 1988 it was 69 percent. Today the census in many hospitals is decreasing because of overcapacity. Because we have become used to it—and vainly expect someone else to "take care of it"—we are becoming increasingly desensitized to the system's waste, abuse, and negligence.

What can be done about these problems?

I believe that the solutions center on the recognition of some hard realities and the application of common sense: a more focused approach on the effectiveness of health care; concentration on cost-effectiveness; more professional administration and a shift to a more pragmatic set of measurable outcomes—treating patients with the best care possible—and seeing the doctor as the patient's friend, not as the hospital's target for its appeal. The monitoring of medical providers is needed to grade the better performers and eliminate the poor ones, and we need hospitals, physicians, specialists, and medical laboratories that are readily available to the American public.

A particular source of the problem is the attitude of American industry, which, in fact, has a vast stake in health care but allows its influence to be wasted and misdirected. If only some of those wasted billions could be recovered and deployed in needy medical projects and services for our people, what boons they might provide!

In 1988 and 1989, General Motors Corporation spent more than $3 billion on medical expenses, 30 percent more than in 1987 and more than it earned from operations. Southern New England Telephone in 1987 spent close to $40 million on such expenses, 14 percent more than in 1986 and more than double the amount of five years ago. Two years ago, Aetna Life and Casualty Company estimated that it would spend $900 million on health care for its present and future retirees. The sum astounded corporate leaders who had never before calculated that particular liability. Nor had most other companies.

And what has made the sums especially onerous is a new accounting rule that requires companies to include their future retiree health care expenses in their current financial reports—while the employees are still working. This rule will tend to reduce corporate net worth—its assets versus its liabilities. The net effect will be to reduce corporate profits since the increase in annual liability will be recorded as a current operating expense. As one executive responsible for health benefits marketing at a major insurance company has said, "The vast majority of employers are in a wait-and-see mode. They know there is going to be a big problem from what they have learned but they don't know what to do about it."

I am convinced that control of health care costs—perhaps the linchpin in the entire system—can only be managed through a partnership among the medical providers, hospitals, physicians, and nursing homes, and the insurers, government, business, and employees. Each has a critical role to play in eliminating the cost-versus-efficiency trap our medical system has fallen into. The following are some of my recommendations:

◆ At a time when 44 percent of all health care costs come from hospitals, providers cannot remain aloof from the problem. Many experts are calling for limitations on a physician's prerogative to order costly procedures. "You cannot have unfettered decision-making by physicians and you must control their expenditures," said Dr. William Roper, chief of the Health Care Financing Administration.

◆ Corporations, because they are directly or indirectly paying medical bills, should focus this clout, either by negotiating directly or empowering their insurers to bring pressure to bear on their behalf. Small- and medium-sized companies are not too small to have an impact if they band together and utilize existing medical networks negotiated by insurers.

3. National Health Expenditures
Hospital Care

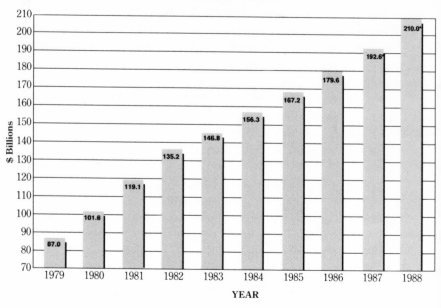

Source: Chart prepared by U.S. Healthcare. Data from U.S. Health Care Financing Administration, *Health Care Financing Review,* summer 1987.

* Estimated.

◆ Insurers must provide the managed-care expertise that corporations demand. They must utilize all their resources to expedite the claims process while conducting tough negotiations, create case management systems that actually work, and pull the pieces together to ensure quality and efficiency. Equally important is the evolution of physicians, hospitals, and most medical procedures—developing algorithms of medical procedures in quantitative terms.

4. National Health Expenditures
Physician's Services

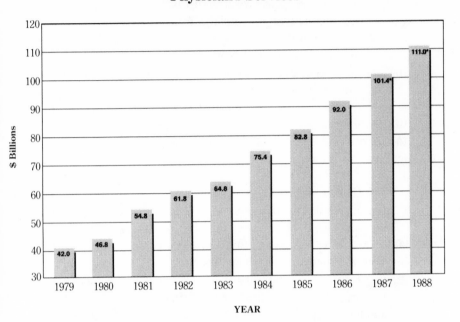

Source: Chart prepared by U.S. Healthcare. Data from U.S. Health Care Financing Administration, *Health Care Financing Review,* summer 1987.

   * Estimated.

◆ Employees who have the most to gain from a more efficient medical delivery system must share the burden of change. A fifteen-year study by the Rand Corporation indicates that the best way to curb overutilization of health care is to shift more financial burden to employees. And employers should offer economic incentives to employees to utilize the best health networks and to be more aggressive about the new programs and understand that they are not sacrificing quality if they can get it by switching from one program to another.

◆ Above all, the entire system must become oriented to functioning in a competitive marketplace. A cost-and-quality equation should govern choice of the medical provider. I do not believe that Americans want a government-run health care system. Not trusting anyone to control such a vital service, they want a pluralistic system with choices. Nevertheless, we know that eventually the cost of health care forces all industrialized nations to organize their health care systems. The United States is no exception, and the inevitable results of a failure to police the private system will lead to government control.

If medicine is eventually organized and we have to surrender our system of private practitioners, we will lose something of inestimable value. U.S. Healthcare, for one, is closely bound to the support of these private practitioners because, after years of working with primary care physicians, we and most successful health maintenance organizations have found that it is the model that really works. The doctor, paid ahead of time, is free to concentrate on helping the patient, and the company is saved endless and costly reviews of individual services.

I believe that the best choice is a well-run, fiscally sound venture involving private medicine, and businesses and employees who pay for the services.

Obviously, I intend to be very candid in this book. The unfolding situation in the American health care system deserves nothing less. We have everything to gain from cleansing the waste, inefficiency, and abuses from our system and nothing to lose from doing so.

The self-correcting ability of our society has been demonstrated again and again, and we can be confident that it can also be applied to our health care system—if we courageously take the steps and means necessary to accomplish this. Capitalism, competition, and education diverted to all segments of our health care delivery system can work.

CHAPTER TWO

Fantasy and Reality in Our $600 Billion Health Care System

In the vast expanse of our $600 billion health care system, there is currently one overarching fantasy: the belief that large insurance companies, large Blue Cross plans, large pharmaceutical companies, and big government organizations have the power and capacity to solve all health care problems. Size has been equated with an endless capability. All of these organizations, according to this popular conception, contain the ability to spend and lose large amounts of money when it comes to providing adequate and efficient health service.

Sadly, the organizations themselves have not only subscribed to but have fostered the fantasy. And when it produced the inevitable, poor results, in desperation they grasped at a variety of lifelines, such as the discount fee-for-service preferred-provider organizations, particularly Medicare, the largest of the PPOs, which is generally considered a gigantic failure. The desperation also led to the giant company that thinks it can be in the health care business itself. General Motors Corporation for three years tried to operate a

PPO with large financial losses, which in 1987 exceeded $500 million. But with every fantasy there is the ultimate bitter reality, and GM has tasted it. After numerous consultants paraded through GM's offices, the giant automaker is now forced to rely upon a small number of experienced health care managers, primarily physicians, to set up standards for quality and quantity in health care. What, one must ask, took so long? And how productively could that money have been used elsewhere?

But that fantasy is only the beginning. There are many more pervading fantasies accompanied by their reverse side, reality, which determine the real scope and shape of our national health care problem.

Many of the plans that pass themselves off as managed health care plans are little more than window dressing for discount fee-for-service indemnity-type insurance plans. In a recent study for the Blue Cross plans in managed health care, Booz, Allen, and Hamilton, the management consultants, criticized their ability to generate and operate true managed health care programs. Blue Cross and Blue Shield HMOs need to focus on getting better as well as bigger. This is also true of the major indemnity insurance companies because their traditional mind-set represents a very basic indemnity thought process. The inevitable result is that such companies are very good at passing along rate increases to their clients. In addition, most major clients have looked upon the insurance company as their advisor or consultant. Somehow, however, it seems that the more the insurance company processes, the more it earns and the more it costs the client organization.

Unfortunately, our huge health care system is actually a fragmented industry composed of many parasitic organizations that feed off the payers of health care. Needless to say, the practice of health care is very dependent upon the payers. As a result, the way in which medicine is practiced and delivered is directly related to the way in which it is paid for. The result is a boom in health care costs.

Another myth is that the payers—in this case, insurance companies and patients—have much to say about the outcome and quality of the product they are paying for. This is not true in fact. In every other segment of our economy, the buyer has at least the opportunity to inspect and reject a product before delivery. But in health care, when it comes to approving what we pay for, it is a fantasy world indeed. We should screen physicians and hospitals, and carefully review outcomes, but quantity many times passes for quality.

In the past, the payer has had little to say about the quality of the health care he is financing. Besides, since patients are generally not knowledgeable about what they need and what should be done, they rely solely upon the doctor's reputation. But reputation is often spread by word of mouth and based upon personality and the quality of advertising and public relations rather than the quality of the health care delivered. In many ways, the individual seeking medical help is left to flounder in a vacuum, uncertain about whom he or she can go to.

In a related problem, psychiatrists and psychologists schedule their treatment sessions based upon the reimbursement that they expect to receive from the insurance carrier, not necessarily upon the intensity of the need of the patient. They are not alone. Podiatrists, for example, have learned to treat an individual patient as ten patients, each toe representing a billing opportunity. They can and do present a bill for each phalange and each tarsal and metatarsal! It is not uncommon for an insurance company to see a bill for office procedures from a podiatrist in excess of $500 or $600. In fact, many times, podiatric bills rival those for cardiac surgery. At times, insurers will receive bills of $4,000, $5,000, or even $6,000 for podiatric office procedures. We have created an environment in which providers have become better at billing than they are at practicing their craft.

In many university hospitals, the size of the accounting department sometimes rivals that of the medical staff itself. The irony of this is that many times hospitals will announce that they are losing money, while the profits from individual departments are kept separate from the funds and books of the hospital as a whole. There are university hospitals in large cities that allow accounts under the supervision of department heads to run from $5 million to $50 million in surplus, generated over the years in which the department head was allowed discretionary spending authority.

Some university and other large hospitals have set up corporations and subsidiaries that in many cases are losing money. The losses of these corporations and subcorporations are then integrated into the losses of the total hospital; the financial people then attempt to pass this on to the third-party payer as real hospital costs. Often the corporations' activities only tangentially involve the hospital and may represent the investment and diversification attempted by well-paid corporation executives.

The fantasy is that somehow all this will either get straightened out or go away, while in fact the federal government is now strapped with $150 billion a year of debt payment on a $2 trillion debt and cannot—and should not—get further involved in paying for health care. Medicare and Medicaid are adding greatly to the cost burdens of the federal government. Fourteen percent of the government's operating cost today is eaten up by debt payment.

The reality of this Catch-22 in health care costs is that discipline and correction are necessary in the medical marketplace and competition must be the governing factor. Of course, when it comes to physician or hospital fees and the posture of third-party payers, the issues can become quite heated. Control of health care costs is viewed as an infringement on the fee-for-service sector, which, I submit, remains one of the last monopolies in our society. Battle lines are drawn. Each side espouses its own data, studies supporting them are developed, and the debate continues. The intensity of this conflict is also fueled by medical journals and magazines that develop a one-sided attitude aimed to please and placate their subscribers. It isn't unusual at all to find in such a publication an issue in the debate distorted and blown out of proportion to soothe the egos and further the economic interests of the magazine's subscribers.

There are idealists who might believe that such abuses, in an area of such great public benefit, will eventually be corrected or removed by public or governmental pressure. Obviously, this hasn't happened, but somehow the optimism of such individuals prevents the public from perceiving the issue as a high priority. We must forget voluntary self-correction. Public exposure and, to a certain extent, the government must begin to exert pressure on the industry. Health containment efforts usually end up in defeat because hospital accounting staffs and physicians usually can find loopholes to get price increases. Take, for example, the DRG system, the diagnosis-related group, which was hailed as a new vehicle auguring for cost saving and efficiency. In the first year of the DRG, there was indeed a reduction in health care costs. Then, as hospitals acquired the appropriate software and learned to work and even alter the DRG recognition and identification factors, diagnoses were changed and DRGs became just another method of maximizing reimbursement.

How much of our health care delivery system is warranted and productive? I think that stronger controls and more selective access are the answer to the explosion of services and the maximizing of health care reimbursement. I am convinced, too, that the reduction of unnecessary health care in itself would reduce our national health bill by more than 20 percent.

The reality is that even though we spend more money than other socially developed countries, we get less for our health care dollar. We spend almost $2,000 per capita on health services compared to about $700 per capita in Great Britain and about $300 per capita in Greece. But all three countries have approximately the same mortality and morbidity rates. People in Great Britain, in fact, have a longer life expectancy and a lower mortality rate. I think it is nothing less than a national disgrace that we spend more than $2 billion a day on health care while 37 million Americans do not have access to health care. The dramatic growth of health care in recent years requires a deep examination of what we really get for our expenditures and a comparison with other countries.

In the traditional indemnity type of health insurance programs, there are more uncovered services that require greater out-ofpocket expenditures but which offer almost complete freedom to select where and from whom the care will be provided. But even with this so-called freedom, the statistics for the outcome of dollars spent for freedom of choice do not yield better health care results.

On the contrary, studies have shown that a managed health care system provides health results as good as, if not better than, the freedom-to-choose, fee-for-service system. The real waste in the system is becoming increasingly noted by experts. Robert H. Brook, of the Rand Corporation, estimates that about one-fifth, or about $120 billion, of medical care in the U.S. is unnecessary. Sidney M. Wolfe, who heads the Public Citizen Health Research Group founded by Ralph Nader, the consumer activist, said that it is unnecessary and incompetent care that contributes to the deaths of more than 200,000 Americans a year. And so in the midst of plenty there is famine. What is undoubtedly the most damning study to be furnished so far was the Federal Mortality Report issued in 1986 and 1987, which suggested that many Medicare patients were dying because they went to hospitals that provided below-average care.

So much for fantasy and reality in our health care system. I will continue to elaborate on both throughout this book. Meanwhile, I want to proceed to hospitals, which in many cases are proving inadequate to their important task. There are notable exceptions, of course, but their example simply dramatizes the lack of quality, service, and management that prevails in many hospitals throughout our nation.

CHAPTER ♦ THREE

Hospitals' Ills

In a typical colony of social bees, the drones and workers revolve about the queen bee. All the priorities and action are based on perpetuating her preeminent role.

If we compare the typical hospital with the buzzing environment of the honeycomb—and there are probably more than a few similarities—we find a difference when it comes to the motivating individual. It isn't the patient, who it should be. Instead, it's the physician, who it shouldn't be. And, as a result, all the priorities and actions of these giant institutions are out of kilter.

Most of us would rather not be patients in a hospital. We don't even like to visit them. Starting with the admissions procedures in most hospitals, the priorities are wrong, and the individual is promptly dehumanized. The admissions clerk or nurse is more interested in learning if you are insured and by whom than whether you are really sick, what is wrong with you, and what should be done. Frequently, a nonemergency patient has a long wait and sits miserably until attended.

One might even say that once the hospital patient is under care, he or she has fewer rights than residents of correctional facilities. At least prisoners have the right to receive visitors during reasonable hours, but a hospital patient sometimes has no such rights. In fact, visiting hours are scheduled at the convenience of the staff. Visitors are sometimes asked to leave even though a visit by a loved one or friend might be more uplifting and appropriate than another blood test.

What happens when a patient's insurance carrier wants to review the case to ensure that appropriate service is being provided? Very often, the carrier is denied access even when the patient requests it. In short, the patient's normal civil rights are denied. Upon entering the hospital, he becomes isolated and subject to the rules and regulations of the hospital, which are not always based on the patient's best interests.

And then there's the question of hospitals' scheduling of more serious matters. Why must a patient be awakened in the middle of the night, or even asked to enter the hospital the night before, so that they may be "prepped" for early morning surgery? The fact is that physicians have for many years performed surgery or visited hospitalized patients in a nonsurgical case in the morning so that they could conduct their office hours in the afternoon. Early morning surgery has nothing to do with any specific biological or clinical factors but with the convenience of the professionals. Why can't patients be operated on on Saturday or Sunday, since the hospital is open and all services are available at that time? This procedure would be cost-effective and prevent a surgical patient from having to wait over a weekend for a necessary operation. Hospitals have never developed their policies and procedures around the patient or treated the community as its customers. Instead, it is all too clear that the physician is the only real customer of any concern to the hospital.

One can't help wondering if this was always so. The history of hospitals shows that they were established to meet the needs of society, and developed along with the growth of national populations. While it is true that hospitals were for the most part primitive, utilitarian facilities, from the first separate institutions for the care and shelter of the sick in the first century A.D., their evolution was always based on healing. Those first Roman hospitals were used for slaves, later for freemen. Throughout the Roman Empire, the establishment of military hospitals inevitably led to the establishment of those for civilians. A dimension of benevolence grew under the influence of Christianity, leading to the first openly public institutions.

During the Middle Ages, the trend to reserve social institutions for the ill also grew in the Middle East where the Muslim rulers and public officials built them in the urban centers. The first rose in the ninth century in Baghdad, followed by two others. The third was a teaching hospital with a staff of twenty-five physicians. In Islamic countries, there were thirty-four hospitals, generally well operated and organized, reflecting the advanced state of contemporary medical practice in those lands. In a Cairo hospital opened in 1283, there were sections for patients with febrile diseases, sections for the wounded, for those with eye diseases, and for women. A director headed a staff of physicians that supervised both male and female nurses.

During the medieval years, monastic orders in the West helped to develop more beneficent hospitals, providing examples for the later, secular institutions. Then hospitals were fostered by the popes and by knightly orders that rose during the Crusades and the holy wars. Eventually, European cities founded hospitals and wealthy burghers and merchants contributed sums to develop and expand them. But it was the medieval European hospitals attended by monks and nuns in the thirteenth and fourteenth centuries that created the model for a foundation of hospitals, followed by the secular community in fifteenth-century France, which established an organized hospital administration and elected a hospital director who appointed his own staff. By the end of the fifteenth century, Europe already had a network of hospitals. More than 750 hospitals were functioning in England alone by that time, and on the Continent there was a similar growth.

Over the next four centuries, the need to minister to community health increased as the towns of Europe grew and urban clusters sprouted. And as social classes became more distinct, the need for care for those at the bottom of the order also grew. Hence, in the sixteenth and seventeenth centuries, hospitals in England and France became places for the sick, the old, and the very poor. Locally financed and administered by a community, parish, or town, they eventually came under the control of a larger government body and ultimately of national authorities. It became obvious that the burden of maintaining an ever-growing hospital—and meeting its social demands—required attention and funds from bodies with greater resources.

General hospitals, the forerunner of today's great health complexes, began in mid-seventeenth-century France as a combination of hospital and almshouse. Even in a time of revolt, a growing sense of obligation to the poor and the afflicted was being felt in France and throughout Europe.

As the number and capacity of hospitals grew in Europe and in the United States, the English style of hospital construction and administration was slowly being emulated in the United States. London's general hospitals were overcrowded and administrators coped, often in vain, with both financial and administrative burdens. The pressure for more beds, especially for the more difficult diseases and afflictions, eventually led to the rise of special hospitals, such as those for smallpox, venereal diseases, and mental disorders. In the English colonies, there developed the same trend toward general and specialized hospitals.

The first American general hospital, the Pennsylvania Hospital, opened its doors in 1751 and the second, the New York Hospital, rose in 1791. But the slow pace of urbanization in the new country also kept the number of hospitals low through much of the nineteenth century. And financial and administrative burdens hampered the American hospitals as much as they did the English. In both the new country and the old, the involvement of private institutions and individuals grew over the years, creating a tradition of private support that continues today.

The present great American hospitals, which evolved over the last 125 years, were at first ineffective in controlling the diseases that swept through a city and the surrounding countryside every few years. Because knowledge of diseases was lacking, the public felt that the hospital was a place to be feared and avoided. But, fortunately, the advent of bacteriology and the breakthroughs of first antiseptic and then aseptic surgery changed that attitude, propelling the hospital into a new, credible role. In fact, by the turn of the twentieth century, the aura of the hospital as a center of social good had grown markedly as a result of not only the development of asepsis but the arrival of X-ray technology, laboratory diagnosis methods, and various therapeutic techniques. Hospitals in the United States also emulated European ones by becoming teaching schools, where doctors and nurses benefited from the on-site learning provided by the growing number of patients.

As the credibility of the hospital rose in the minds of the public, admissions grew dramatically, fostered by the realization that a sick person was better off in a hospital. In 1873 there were 146,472 admissions to American hospitals. By 1945 the annual figure had risen to 16,257,406, and by 1961 to 25,474,000. The increase was a direct reflection of the nation's population growth, but it also affirmed the increasing importance of the hospital as a social necessity. The admissions growth over the subsequent years necessitated the addition of adjunct services, including those provided by psychiatrists, social workers, and home-careists, not to mention the need for a much more complex administrative infrastructure. But these changes made the hospital facility too complex and led to a communications lag, excessive costs, and a reconsideration of hospital administration.

Such problems led to the appearance of the hospital administrator, who would become a key player on the medical stage as well as in the development and explosive growth of voluntary advance payments for hospital care, new standards for hospital quality, and a new, important role for government in regard to the building and financing of hospitals. Whereas at the beginning of the twentieth century most American hospitals were private or voluntary and few were government-supported, since the mid-1920s, tax-supported hospitals have increased sharply in number and taxes have also been used to pay private hospitals to care for people on public assistance.

The number of American hospitals grew dramatically with the Hospital Survey and Construction Act of 1946, known as the Hill-Burton Act. Initially providing for a $3 million appropriation to survey hospital needs throughout the states and $75 million to build government and nongovernment hospitals during a five-year period, and amended a number of times over the next few decades, the Hill-Burton Act has accounted for a vast amount of new facilities, hospital beds, and general medical services.

But if the growth of hospital services has been dramatic, the ills of hospitals, too, have become noteworthy, centering on social, economic, and political conflicts. Have hospitals become too big a business to carry out their traditional commitment to serve "the afflicted, the poor and the old," as their early sponsors wished? Are hospital administrators, who used to be called "hospital super-intendents" before they expressed a preference for the more euphemistic title, failing to carry out their commitment to supervise a socially responsive institution? The "presidents" of hospitals sometimes forget their real calling and wear their title with cold aloofness. It seems that the answer to these questions is yes, and hospitals must reconsider their history and return to their tradition of social service.

Yet most hospitals continue to gear their schedules and marketing efforts to the physician who will help fill their beds and maintain a high patient population. Many hospital administrators are concerned with little else. If the hospital is filled and running at 90 percent occupancy, the administrator is certain to be rewarded for doing a good job. Physicians who contribute to a high census by having many patients are sought after and even pampered as "cash cows." Hospital administrators cater to these heavy hitters and schedule operating-room time for them on a priority basis.

These privileges, unfortunately, are not extended because the physicians produce the best surgical results or practice the most cost-effective medicine. Like the superproductive physician he favors, the typical hospital administrator may not be judged by his or her colleagues for the quality of the institution but for its bed capacity. Often we hear an administrator described as the head of "a five-hundred-bed, tertiary care facility." Larger hospitals carry more prestige. And at a time when an occupied hospital bed can command as much as $2,000 to $3,000 a day, the physician-producers are much prized. Conversely, those physicians who spend their time and energy treating patients in a more service-oriented or quality outpatient setting, or even in their offices, will continue to lose prestige and influence in the health care industry. But those physicians who are responsible for the most admissions, who use consultants most frequently, and who order the largest battery of tests and procedures will continue to be the most influential, the most sought after, even though they are steering the course of medicine in a direction contrary to the public interest.

Hospital superintendents used to live at the hospital and were responsible for making certain that it was clean and that laundry, food, and other services were properly maintained. However, since the advent of the Hill-Burton bill and the Medicare law of 1965, there has developed a need for a variety of administrators: facility managers, accountants, reimbursement specialists, and others. Administrators became a new breed, with master's degrees in hospital administration from recognized colleges and universities. They were looked upon as prizes for hospitals, especially if they also became reimbursement specialists. They attained a reputation for financial acumen if they could bring in a glowing bottom line rather than praise as an administrator of a quality facility.

Who are the administrators? It seems to vary from city to city. In Boston, for example, many are M.D.'s, while in other cities, such as Philadelphia, hardly any hospital administrators have graduated from medical school, but have business-education backgrounds. The difference in background stems from the particular hospital's

tradition, the composition of its board, and other indigenous factors, such as the political complexity between the hospital administration and the physician's staff.

   The irony of the situation is that making money in the hospital
business became relatively easy once Medicare was off and running. All one had to do was find a decent location. Financing was
easy. Reimbursement was guaranteed. And all that was needed to
get a profitable hospital going was to find an ambitious hospital
administrator, a senior financial officer, and a head nurse. Even the
financial officer's job was facilitated by the inevitable visits from
computer software suppliers who recognized a need in hospitals
and accordingly packaged ready-made software programs to help
maximize reimbursement and to operate all business functions.
Naturally, the software company's salesmen were go-getters. They
eagerly notified the administrator that if such and such a software
package is used, "your reimbursement will increase by so much
and therefore the package or service in essence is a self-financing
one." Nothing, in other words, to worry about.

   Wasn't society aware of this situation?

   This question has been asked before—in fact, it may be asked in
every chapter of this book because I feel that public awareness of
the problems of our health care system may make all the difference
in the world. One can only assume that the public either doesn't
know, is distracted by other things—or, least likely, doesn't care.

   However, I think it is the misdirected goals of the typical American hospital, accompanied by high costs and the lack of quality
service, that demonstrate how our society condones and even
accepts "cheating" in our health care system. Helped by the major
public accounting firms in this country, hospitals contrive to
squeeze out more money from the federal government and third-
party payers than they actually deserve or can adequately account
for. Their mind-set is that if they are questioned and found to have
inflated their bills, they will return the money. But the hard fact is
that many get away with it. In so doing, they cost the United States
and its economy hundreds of millions of dollars in unnecessary
health care costs.

And one must question the ethics of the big accounting firms that, after helping the hospitals inflate their bills, then turn around to the payers and try to sell them "antidote computer software." What for? So that the payer can uncover the situations where the unscrupulous hospital is getting more than it should in payment. Take the DRG system, the diagnosis-related group, mentioned in the previous chapter. Or the per case method of payment adopted by Medicare and other payers. If certain procedures are listed in a specific order, or if the hospital can get the physician to indicate that a problem became "complicated" or was accompanied by a "complication," then the hospital can receive much more payment than it would otherwise be entitled to. Since most cases involve subjective judgments, they can be easily supported if the physicians or nurses document their findings in the medical records. Respected consulting firms and hospitals even conduct seminars throughout the country to train employees and physicians how to cheat those who pay the medical bills.

Both Blue Cross and Medicare calculated all the possible costs that could be incurred in a hospital and included them in the reimbursement package. But hospitals managed to justify their coverage in a variety of creative ways. They misrepresented their work for many years, well into the late 1980s, until the advent of the DRG and its more precise accounting methods.

Why is there a constant gap between costs and charges? First, it seems worth repeating that in many American hospitals the business office staff is second in size only to the nursing department. The number of accountants employed by that office may soon rival the number of physicians who work in a hospital. Complex formulas were developed to justify costs by hospitals, and their itemizations did not coincide with those developed by Blue Cross and Medicare.

Also, for a long time Medicare didn't seem to care what it was charged as long as it was appropriately billed. Many times, I have learned, when auditors from Medicare visited a hospital, the accounting department was told, in effect, "We'll pay you if you apply it to a certain, recognized category." Costs, in other words, became a classification game, and when those of us in the managed health care business came to negotiate with hospitals, they would tell us, "Well, Medicare pays us and these are our costs."

I am convinced that many hospitals don't even know what their costs are. Through the years, they have been so busy calculating reimbursement formulas that they have forgotten what their true expenses are. In 1990 it isn't uncommon to see a patient's costs running from $1,000 to $10,000 a day. And it isn't uncommon to see billings for a patient's stay running to several hundred thousand dollars. What is even more exasperating is to see a bill for an elderly patient reaching $100,000, $150,000, and even $200,000. The knowledge that the patient would die anyway did not stop the hospital from offering the patient the most expensive treatment.

Many of us in the managed health care field have seen cases in which the billing system dictated what should be done to the patient the moment he entered the hospital. We have all heard the stories about the twenty-dollar aspirin tablet; as the maximization of reimbursement continues, it is only a question of how long the ingenuity of accounting procedures will enable the hospitals to rip off the American public.

Is it any wonder that a 1988 survey of 1,400 general acute-care community hospitals found that administrators of 700 of the hospitals feared that their institutions would be forced to close in the next five years because of financial problems, including government curbs on Medicare payments?

Why then, if hospitals have learned to maximize reimbursement, are so many hospitals in financial trouble?

1. Hospitals have poor cost accounting systems. They don't know their real costs.
2. Hospitals have been "gaming" the system so long they believe their own rhetoric.

Raymond J. Cisneros, of the accounting firm Touche Ross and Company, said in the *Washington Post,* "The fact that so many hospitals anticipate failure is even more dramatic when one realizes that 150 hospitals have already closed in the past two years."

The Medicare system, attempting to curb costs, started a prospective payment system in 1983. This sets a fixed payment in advance for every hospital stay and normally doesn't pay more, regardless of how many days the patient remains there or what tests or services the patient gets. And Congress's setting of fixed payments has not kept pace with inflation as both houses and the White House have sought to reduce the federal deficit. As a result, almost 70 percent of the administrators responding to the Touche Ross survey, most of them representing rural hospitals, said that their hospitals' incomes have fallen since the advent of the new Medicare system.

There can be little doubt that in the majority of hospitals, costs can be contained even with lower Medicare payment if traditionally wasteful and inefficient policies are ended. I will discuss hospitals further in subsequent chapters on physicians, HMOs, and insurers.

CHAPTER ◆ FOUR

The Management of Health Care: Who Does What and How Well?

If hospitals can be likened to a beehive, think of total American health care as a huge, multifauceted pipeline. It has six faucets: the "Blues" (Blue Cross and Blue Shield), the HMOs (health maintenance organizations), the PPOs (preferred-provider organizations), the indemnity insurance companies, and of course the government in the form of Medicare and Medicaid. Each is a payment facility. Sometimes they gush freely. Other times fitfully. In any case, they need to be fixed.

All civilized societies recognize that health care costs have to be insured by a third party—the government, an insurance company, or another entity which bears the risk. In our society, we have a worrisome third-party-payer mentality.

The purpose of this chapter is to provide some insight into how these programs define their mission and how they operate, and to allow the reader to appraise their effectiveness in controlling health costs.

THE "BLUES"

The Blue Cross plans operate in many parts of the United States as independent entities linked by a central organization, Blue Cross of America, based in Chicago. In many states, there are three or more Blue Cross plans functioning separately. In Pennsylvania, the home state of my company, there is a plan called Independence Blue Cross, which operates in the metropolitan Philadelphia area and is really the entity providing hospital insurance. There is also a Blue Shield plan that covers various parts of the state and which insures the physician's portion of health care costs, and there are separate Blue Cross plans in Pittsburgh, Harrisburg, and northeastern Pennsylvania.

Usually, the Blue Cross plans themselves insure the hospital portion of payment and the Blue Shield plans insure the physician's portion. In some states, however, there is cooperation and in others open competition, particularly with the advent of new third-party plans such as HMOs. In Pennsylvania this is the case, with Blue Shield operating the Keystone Health Plan and Blue Cross plans operating their own independent HMOs.

It is interesting to note that these nonprofit organizations often own for-profit subsidiaries. It's also noteworthy that the Blue Cross plan in Philadelphia pays its president more than $500,000 in salary and highly rewards its other executives even though in the last two years the plan has shown rather large losses. The Blue Cross plan in Philadelphia has diversified into the HMO business, the utilization review business, and the indemnity insurance business. Moreover, it is dabbling in commercial real estate investment, a remote tangent from the early mission of developing an insurance entity that would provide low-cost hospital insurance for individuals.

Many states have blessed Blue Cross plans with favorable legislation that gives them a discount, such as the 13 percent discount for hospital payments in New York. The Blue Cross boards are often composed of hospital managers, physicians, and a variety of other leaders in the community. The plans' rates have risen as fast as any consumer-based services in the country. So I believe one must question whether or not Blue Cross plans are merely a means of providing payment to hospitals. Research has shown that when Blue Cross plans venture into the HMO business and compete in the open market, their effectiveness leaves much to be desired. The consulting firm Booz, Allen, and Hamilton has criticized their ability to manage health care costs, even in an HMO environment.

The favorable legislation in many states giving Blue Cross plans unmerited discounts on hospital rates has produced an oligopoly in substantial areas of the country where Blue Cross is the major insurer for large numbers of people. I believe that Blue Cross has contributed to the delinquency and unnecessary extra costs of health care. Even with their hospital discounts, the Blue Cross plans in 1988 lost an estimated $1 billion while rate increases for individuals and small groups have mounted 50 to 60 percent per year in recent years.

Blue Cross plan ratings are variable because different groups can be and are rated individually. Because of that and because of the variety of plans, it is very difficult to compare costs for an employer or an individual. Another reason is the Blue Cross mentality, which views the hospital as its client, shaping its cost structure and policies to benefit the hospital rather than the employer or the insured. Kansas City Blue Cross recently appealed to its hospitals for a cash infusion. The financially troubled plan reasoned that they had been the hospitals' friend.

An exception is the St. Louis Blue Cross, in which Blue Cross and Blue Shield have been merged into a single entity. This in itself has led to greater efficiency and cooperation. The management has also made a major commitment to building an alternate, managed, health care system. Another benefit of the merger is the strong potential for a new breed of Blue Cross manager. The plan president and a board of informed members are establishing reasonable targets of accountability in rates and profitability.

The reverse of the St. Louis example is Blue Cross of Greater Philadelphia. The City of Brotherly Love is blessed with a Blue Cross plan that competes with Blue Shield, competes with itself and, while claiming special status for public service, has used subscriber money for a Veterans Stadium superbox and an expensive Center City office building project. The Philadelphia management also recently sought a change in the plan's bylaws that would have removed public representation from its board and left power squarely in the hands of its "corporate" managers.

It is worth noting that the Blue Cross plans in New York, Pittsburgh, and Philadelphia started as nonprofit entities for the purpose of selling low-cost hospital insurance. But this mission took a new course under the control of individuals who, in my view, seem to aspire more to assume the mantle of senior corporate officers than wear the nonprofit cloak of public service. Profits and the good life were always very much there under the surface.

Certain Blue Cross plans have built large offices and splurged on office equipment and space. Their original raison d'être seems to have escaped them, and one cannot help but wonder how far these individuals can carry their self-interest beyond that of a democratically run for-profit or nonprofit organization.

It's as important for the Blues to evaluate their operation as it is for every other institution in the health care field at a time of rapidly escalating costs. As we enter the 1990s, management of health care is rapidly becoming vital for all insurance entities; those who do not embrace some sort of managed health care will be so parasitized by a runaway medical delivery system that either the rates will reach impossible heights or it will be necessary to depart the business.

Why are we facing a crisis? At present the hospital community receives income from the federal government through Medicare, from private insurance companies, and from HMOs. Medicare has set a limit on its rate of increase of between 3 and 4 percent a year. This means that the hospitals will inevitably have to shift costs to the private insurance companies and the HMOs. But since the

HMOs also very aggressively negotiate rates, this means that the cost shift will be left to the residual of those companies that have no managed health care or those that pay charges.

Therefore, it is conceivable that in a shrinking market where there is pure indemnity pay or self-insurance that pays full charges, hospitals will raise their fees as high as they possibly can to try and recoup what they envision as the shortfall in their budgets. Hospitals are aggressive and imaginative in their ability to maximize billings to those customers who pay full fee-for-service.

HMOS

When federally qualified HMOs were created through the enactment in 1972 of Public Law 93-222, the idea behind the government's funding and sponsorship was to inject a new wave of competition into the health care arena. I believe that most students of this piece of legislation will grant that the effort has been very successful. It helped to bring about not only government-sponsored HMOs but also privately sponsored HMOs which themselves brought new competition. The HMOs and their activities resulted in a reduction of the length of hospital stays because they modified the conduct of physicians who practice within their contract. These physicians have accepted both the medical and financial responsibility for their patients and utilize laboratory services and other outpatient services better because they are unlimited in the HMO program.

The HMOs have their problems but on the whole have made remarkable strides, as is evident by their strong market penetration. Margo L. Vignola, an analyst for Salomon Brothers, the investment bankers, made these points in a May 1988 research study on HMOs: "Prepaid health care, commonly termed health maintenance organizations (HMOs), provides a unique blend of insurance and service delivery. Unlike indemnity insurance,

HMOs impose no payment or deductible charge—all care is covered by a monthly premium. The HMO company in turn contracts for or arranges for medical treatment either through salaried physicians or capitated payment to providers. Members must use these providers to assure coverage of expenses. In addition, HMOs have also traditionally sought to minimize the use of costly services such as hospital care."

Vignola added that despite the wrenching changes affecting HMOs in the 1987–88 period, industry trends and characteristics remain "strikingly unchanged."

Continuing, she said: "Although the rate of enrollment growth slowed in 1987, HMOs still posted solid gains for the year. Through September, membership reached 28.8 million, up by 11.9 percent from year-earlier levels. HMOs now claim about 10 percent of the nation's non-Medicare population. HMOs' market share and enrollment have more than doubled since 1983 when they first became publicly traded entities."

The most effective HMOs are those that share the risks with hospitals and providers such as U.S. Healthcare. These programs are funded by a payment mechanism called "capitation." Simply stated, capitation is a negotiated or predetermined amount of money which is paid bimonthly to the medical providers for services. This in essence does away with the piecework type of billing and also removes the maximizing of reimbursement so prevalent in the medical community. Capitation has evolved over the last sixteen years. There are modifications of the capitation of payment whereby an individual-practice-association corporation, composed of primary care and family physicians, is formed and the insuring entity pays either a fee for services or a discount to its subscribing providers. But this form of payment is usually not successful.

The HMO payment mechanism leads to and accommodates three types of organization. One is the staff model, whereby physicians and medical providers are on staff and are usually paid a salary. Another type, the group model, occurs when physicians form into groups and contract to provide services. Kaiser Permanente in California and Harvard Community Health Care in Boston are examples of such group models. Specialists, hospitals, and ancillary services, such as radiology and laboratory facilities, are included in these arrangements. The groups can and do at times act independently.

Then there are new hybrid groups called PPOs (preferred-provider organizations) and EPOs (employer purchase organizations) that have been formed by the insurance industry and hospitals to create new, competitive health care organizations. In these groups, the pure discount fee-for-service models usually do not work simply because the provider can control the utilization. Thus, if a physician renders services to an insuring entity or company at a 30 to 40 percent discount merely by increasing utilization by one more visit, this practice will obliterate any cost savings.

But I think that as we move into the 1990s the structure of all these plans will be dictated by the marketplace and the practical needs of Americans. As a result, purists who feel that the group model or the staff model or the individual-practice-association model is in itself the sole solution or form are, in my opinion, mistaken. I believe that the hybrids and their modifications are the design of the future. So rather than detailing a historical development of the HMO field, I feel it is of greater importance to the reader to understand that managed health care in itself will remain a permanent part of the American medical delivery system and it is the marketplace that will dictate what forms the HMOs and the PPOs or other managed health care organizations will take. It's my conviction that all indemnity insurance companies and the federal government will adopt managed health care in some form because these structures promise the best economic format.

Incidentally, the largest PPO in the United States is Medicare and it certainly has been far from a success. Managed health care must close the loopholes that allow for maximization of reimbursement.

After all, it is only reasonable that healing our health care system is as much a function of design as need. When we accept the premise that 20 percent of our health care costs are either unnecessary or ineffective, we can then design approaches to change these abuses. Well-run HMOs operate on this premise not by withholding care but by functioning in the belief that appropriate care is both effective and efficient. Those in traditionally managed fee-for-service health care want the public to believe that the more care one gets and the more it costs, the better.

When we consider that several hundred thousand people a year die because of overcare and concentration on fees rather than service and realize that much of this practice is defensive in nature to protect physicians against litigation-prone lawyers, it's not difficult to see the need for change in both thinking and policy.

INDEMNITY INSURANCE COMPANIES

Historically, indemnity insurance companies (e.g., Cigna, Metropolitan, Aetna) provided a wide range of health insurance benefits for which the employer bore no risk beyond the premium payments made on behalf of its employees.

But over time this has changed considerably to the point where the predominant form of insurance at this point is really noninsurance. Several factors have created this evolution.

To begin with, it has been recognized for many years that group insurers serve primarily as providers of services, such as claim handling and administration. In addition, they have provided what amounts to cash-flow management services because they budget expenditures through the payment of monthly premiums. However, unless the employer has been willing to change insurance carriers frequently over the years, it eventually pays the entire cost for the claims of its employees. The employer has also had to pay the administrative expenses of the insurance company in handling those claims and related services and a profit charge for the insurance company. And both the insurer and the employer have long recognized that there is no such thing as a free lunch and that the employer ultimately bears the expense.

For years this arrangement worked with most changes revolving around the form or method in which the premium payment was made. Initially, simple monthly payment with no retrospective analysis of the results was the most common approach. Later came arrangements such as additional-premium clauses, minimum-premium plan arrangements, and, ultimately, administrative-services-only agreements. All of these plans to varying degrees enabled the employer to utilize his funds for longer periods of time in the management of his core business and to pay health costs only as they developed.

These programs received a tremendous developmental push in the 1970s when a number of factors came together to outweigh their administrative difficulties. First, there were very high investment rates available in the marketplace. Employers preferred to hold their own funds and invest them at these attractive rates or plow them back into their business instead of taking the relatively modest rates that most insurance companies were crediting at the time on cash flow.

Second, premium taxation by the states, which is typically 2 percent or more of premium, encouraged the development of programs in which premiums were depressed by financial arrangements that shifted more of the risk to the employer. And third, with the advent of ERISA (the Employee Retirement Income Security Act of 1974), self-insurance programs got a major push as ERISA provided a preexemption from state-mandated benefits for self-insured programs. The combined influence of these factors proved overwhelmingly in favor of self-insured programs for many employers.

But self-defense came to the fore. Most insurers tried to prevent the development of such self-insured programs as these ultimately led to more scrutiny of the insurer's charges, by employers for retention or for administrative expenses and profit. Retention is an actuarial term used to calculate a portion of the profits. Clearly, as companies begin to seek competitive bids for ASO (administrative services only), the scrutiny of expenses and profits can become more intense. Moreover, as these expenses are tangible, the employer often places more importance on them than on potential future benefits and cost savings, which are normally less tangible and less quantifiable. Clients of insurance companies have been more sensitive to service than cost.

Over the years, insurance companies have realized that the employer must pay the full freight for benefits, expenses, and profits and so have really considered their business to be a service industry. The larger insurers have looked for clients who were willing to enter into a long-term relationship and who would hopefully not desert the insurer the first time a deficit was incurred in order not to have it recouped by the company.

And, as an outgrowth of their service-oriented nature, insurance companies have been willing to provide whatever product design and financing mechanism the client desired. They recommend products and services that they believe would best meet the client's needs. However, what the client wants ultimately defines the product. This is a basic premise of many sales organizations, including insurance companies. You can't make a profit if you don't make the sale. Employee benefit officers have become accustomed to using insurance companies and brokers as consultants, not insurance entities.

To my mind, one of the greatest differences in the philosophy of insurance companies versus that of my company, U.S. Healthcare, is that an insurance company is primarily interested in selling business and making a reasonable profit. There has been little interest in managing health care costs and in helping reduce and control the utilization of health care services. But this may be looked upon as a way to increase competitive advantage and increase sales and profits. At USHC, managing health care costs is more of a cause in and of itself, and the goal as well.

It is my belief that appropriately underwritten group health insurance business is no more risky than the business we "write" every day as an HMO. Both pricing mechanisms depend upon a careful and accurate projection of future costs, based upon the evaluation of prior experience and the maintenance of reasonable margins for fluctuation and expense profit levels. It is only when margin levels fluctuate and profits are squeezed or inverted that real problems develop. This has happened repeatedly to indemnity companies and recently to the HMOs as well.

In both fields, companies have reacted to competitive pressures by setting rates in an unduly optimistic manner, causing margins to drop and losses for the companies involved. There is nothing inherently flawed with the price of either the indemnity insurance or HMO coverage. HMO coverage specializes in managing care, whereas indemnity coverage tries to price the risk and experience, with little concern for quality or quantity of care.

Two markets seem to present difficult underwriting for insurance companies. The first one is small groups, generally working for companies with fewer than fifty employees. The employers in this case are often very familiar with the health care situations of their employees, and the administrative burden of shopping for insurance programs frequently is not great. These groups tend to be highly mobile and whenever rate levels are raised or a deficit is experienced, they are prone to move to another insurer before any adjustment in rates or recouping of the deficit can be made.

To date, in our company we have not suffered any exodus of accounts since we do not make any effort to track which accounts represent losses. We do not attempt to adjust their rates nor do we try to recoup deficits. But I believe that we do experience adverse selection because as a federally qualified HMO we cannot exclude members with preexisting conditions. And I think as we move toward class rating and ultimately experience rating in view of the changing market and regulations, we will find, as the indemnity carriers have, that these small cases can be very problematical for us. Small groups are notorious for placing relatives or friends on their books if they are in need of health insurance.

Jumbo accounts are the other difficult category for the insurers to underwrite on a profitable basis. These accounts have been perceived as highly attractive due to their prominence in the marketplace and the presumed prestige of administering a large account. But most companies have found that it is very difficult to gain a profit from them. Competitive pressures are so great that profit margins are often eliminated from the programs in the negotiation process.

Insurance companies continue to evaluate optimistically their opportunities for recouping losses but then get pressured year after year at renewal time into arrangements that provide little or no hope for doing so. Yet they are afraid to lose the account because then they would never recoup the losses and they would also suffer the perceived marketing disadvantage of losing a prestigious account.

It has been my experience that generally companies will only write off a large loss account when the company's overall earnings picture turns so negative that the company just cannot bear to take the losses any further. Through the good times, companies will tolerate moderate losses on large accounts and consider it no more than one of the prices of doing business.

Losses suffered on large and small accounts obviously put pressure on companies to make more money on the medium-sized accounts. These accounts tend to be somewhat more objectively underwritten and are the core of most companies' group insurance business. One can also see why there is a niche for companies such as CNA Insurance that avoid large and small accounts and can, therefore, price medium-sized accounts more competitively.

Group insurance premiums are based on that group's actual experience. Thus, rates are formulated by group underwriters, and are based on a projection of future expenses that is in turn based primarily or exclusively upon experience from the immediate past. For example, the typical group insurance premium-setting formula would indicate that premiums for the last twelve months adjusted to reflect the most current rates are compared with the last twelve months' incurred claims. The latter are the underwriter's best estimate of the company's liability for all physician services received during the period and hospitalizations begun in that period. The incurred claims are multiplied by a trend factor which is projected to approximate the impact of increasing utilization and costs in the next rate period. This calculation yields the projected incurred claims.

These projected incurred claims are increased by a margin factor called an actuarial margin or margin for fluctuation. Typically, the margin factor would be on the order of 12 percent for a 100-employee account and 5 percent for an account of 5,000 employees. This projected incurred claim amount with margin for fluctuation is then increased to cover desired retention charges. Retention charges are composed of expenses, profit margins, and a risk charge.

Of course, expense and profit margins are self-explanatory, but the concept of a risk charge or contribution to a risk pool is not as obvious. In its simplest terms, a risk charge is designed to enable a company to meet its profit objective in an experience-rated environment. When experience rating is utilized, as it typically is, with retrospective analysis on cases that have positive results, the insurer returns all funds in excess of claims, expenses, and desired profit charge. But in cases where there is a negative result, the insurer is left holding the bag.

The net result is that all deficits on cases that have a bad year will come directly out of profits. In order to enable the companies to reach a desired profit goal, a risk charge is assessed, in addition to profit charges, against profitable accounts during the year at a level that is anticipated to offset negative results on accounts that have a bad year. This enables a company to attain the desired profit objective without having to overstate its profit charges in order to reach that goal.

I have deliberately gone into considerable detail at the risk of confusing the unsophisticated reader because I believe it is important to understand how insurers arrive at their charges. Obviously, indemnity companies are clearly more subject to the inflationary pressures in the medical care marketplace than are HMOs. However, recent experience shows more and more that HMOs are not immune from those pressures.

A point to remember is that when we add the benefits of managed care to utilization we teach doctors how to manage the care they deliver better and more appropriately. They begin to operate in that manner for all their patients, not simply for their HMO patients. The indemnity insurers, too, become beneficiaries of HMO management. This trend can be seen in the overall reduction of hospital utilization throughout the United States in the last few years. Of course, the manipulations of the health care system by Medicare also have had a prominent impact on the practice of physicians and hospitals. But I am confident that the spillover from HMO management techniques has also played an important part in the transformation.

To the extent that HMOs have been able to negotiate privileged fees and discounts, they obviously have been able to insulate themselves from some of the forces in the market. It's probably significant to note that insurance companies have not historically neglected this area out of stupidity or laziness but have been crippled by a desire to be national players. But as HMOs have learned, it is difficult to establish national networks and hold them together. Moreover, for many years, indemnity companies were in effect precluded from negotiating fees due to antitrust concerns and unfavorable court decisions.

Experience rating has distinct advantages, particularly that of rating the risk. When you expect a group to have very poor experience, coal miners, for instance, you can set the rate appropriately. And when you expect a group to have favorable experience, again you are able to set the rate in accordance with that expectation and provide the most competitive and appropriate rate for that specific group.

In a community-rating environment such as regulatory agencies have traditionally required of HMOs, you are exposed to significant adverse selection unless your competitors also follow a policy of community rating. To date, we at U.S. Healthcare have not suffered particularly from community rating, as our primary competitors for the employees we tend to enroll are other HMOs that are also community-rated. I believe that class rating for other HMOs has already exposed us to some adverse selection and increased risk as these HMOs tend to quote more attractive rates for groups that are better risks. By attracting those members from our community-rated pool, our remaining overall risk level is increased.

We will have to move toward class rating in 1990 and experience rating in step with our competitors. Otherwise, our results will show significant adverse selection (meaning we could attract members with unusually higher risk than comparable groups) and deteriorating profitability. Community rating rates the entire community, whereas class rating applies to segments with similar characteristics.

The classic rate spiral is almost preventable in this scenario. As you raise the rates and maintain them on a community basis, your competitors who are either in class or experience rating will write a larger number of the favorable risks on which you were previously competitive and your community pool will have somewhat worse experience requiring somewhat higher rates and so on.

Designing a plan to meet the employer's needs is, of course, vital. In the past, significantly more importance has been given to designing products to meet the current needs and desires of the employer. We have had an extremely singular focus that, with the support of section 1310 (the dual-choice mandate) and legislated community rating for HMOs, has made our program extremely successful. The federal mandate section 1310 of Public Law 93-222 mandated employers of twenty-five or more employees to offer HMOs.

However, I believe that environmental and regulatory changes will require us to make adjustments in our product portfolio. Allowing the employer to have more of a role in designing his own plan—e.g., selecting copayment levels and other cost-sharing levels—will play an important role in our future. Products enabling an employer to provide employees with some leakage to an indemnity environment will be the key to allowing us to persuade employers to push larger segments or all of their employees into our managed-care programs.

But as we make such a move, the need to get away from community rating will become increasingly important. Our rates are based upon the type of enrollment we currently experience in head-to-head competition with indemnity plans and other HMOs at the time of open enrollment. As we move to enrolling entire groups, the mix of employees we tend to enroll will significantly change and will require adjustment in our rating. Experience rating will also open a door for us to increase significantly the numbers of employers whom we previously were reluctant to quote. When the rates can be set to consider the risk involved, the underwriting guidelines can be considerably more flexible. In the indemnity world, the concept is much like life insurance. If you can set the rate to reflect the risk, you can insure anything. For example, for someone standing in front of a speeding train who has just requested $100,000 of life insurance, the rate is $100,000 minus ten seconds interest plus expenses and profit!

While experience rating does provide considerably more flexibility, it is also much more demanding for the company. You must be able to provide timely and completely accurate information on the enrollment, premium, and claim history of each experience-rated account. You cannot operate with systems and procedures that do not provide such information, nor can you survive in the experience-rated environment without accurate reporting. Employers are naturally not very sympathetic if you approach them three months after new rates have been set and say, "We just found some more claims that are for your group, and we need to raise your rates." Further still, there is significant impact on staffing needs in the area of underwriting, and increased staff is necessary.

In essence, the experience-rating process requires the procedure used to rate an entire market for each case. Of course, if you have confidence in your systems and automated production reports of experience, this process can be extremely streamlined compared to the process we now go through.

In other words, rating requires, as all other elements of health care management, common sense and practicality in all its phases. We intend to have more to say about this simple but strategic need in later chapters.

CHAPTER ♦ FIVE

The Doctor's
Proliferating Dilemma

Lincolnesque, paternal, and distinguished, former United States Surgeon General C. Everett Koop now plays the role of the nation's tough, crusty, old doctor who tells everyone the way things are no matter who is offended. Whether issuing a stern warning to use condoms to combat AIDS, remonstrating against smoking in public places, or forcing his political superiors to act instead of talk on public health, Dr. Koop has drawn attention to personal health as a commonsense way of life as no one has for years.

As *U.S. News & World Report* said in May 1988, "In reality, plenty of people are after the surgeon general: Cigarette companies, Phyllis Schlafly, Catholic groups, even some Reagan administration officials. But to millions of others, C. Everett Koop is a folk hero, a real-life Dr. Welby swelled to stately proportions, steering America's course through the perils of modern medicine."

In a day and age when the image of the American doctor has been under considerable attack, Dr. Koop's example is a welcome exception, convincing skeptical Americans that there are good, idealistic doctors and surgeons as there were decades ago when many made house calls, didn't charge an arm and a leg, and sincerely worried about patients as though they were family members.

But, to be fair, physicians have many dilemmas facing them nowadays in their everyday practice. There are the dilemmas of a physician's decision-making: what's the best thing for the patient or the doctor, or for the patient or the doctor's hospital? Furthermore, it's necessary for the doctor to protect himself against a malpractice suit.

A doctor is not subject to the checks and balances generated by traditional competitive forces. He can control the frequency of visits. For example, he can tell a patient, "Here is a prescription for medicine to control your blood pressure. I must recheck you in two weeks or else . . ." Or he might say, "This medicine has side effects that can be prevented if detected early. Therefore, I must check you every two weeks."

But an alternative and perhaps better way might be: "Here is a list of reactions to look for. If any of these occur, call me or do the following. . . ."

Again in a case of some cardiac concern, the doctor might say, "I don't think you have heart disease. But there is enough of a possibility that I recommend a series of tests—echocardiogram and stress tests. If negative, we will go on to a thallium stress test and then to an angiogram." But a well-trained clinician can usually make the proper diagnosis without most of these procedures.

There are the dogmatic doctors, too, who might say, "I am the doctor, you're not. I know what is best for you." Unfortunately, most patients agree to these terms—especially when a third party pays.

When a house is being built, the contractor might say, "I build houses, you don't." Yet, how many of us would be so simple as to take that sort of a deal?

Malpractice obviously is the latest dilemma and physicians do get heavily involved in medical malpractice suits. Specialists are flown in from different parts of the country to either defend or help prosecute physicians in a malpractice suit. Malpractice lawyers maintain files of doctors who can quickly be brought in as "hired guns." These physicians are summoned to give expert testimony in a particular medical case, rendering their opinion against that of one of their colleagues. But the same physicians scream when their malpractice insurance premiums are increased.

Simply stated, the physician's dilemma is this: Should physicians hire themselves out to malpractice lawyers for a few pieces of gold or should they take a higher, more ethical viewpoint and decline to become involved in these costly malpractice cases? The fact is that if physicians did not play the expert-testimony game, there is no doubt that insurance costs, and in turn health care costs, could be reduced. Physicians should police their own ranks rather than allow lawyers to create cases that are usually more of a legal circus than of medical merit.

Physicians face pressure from many facets in our society. Their position in society is eroded daily, and their fees are often the topic of discussion and review in the press. This excerpt from *Business Week* magazine (July 11, 1988) is a perfect example.

There's No Quick Cure for High Doctor Bills

The next phase of the medical cost containment era is about to begin. First the federal government put hospital charges under the knife. Later private insurers joined in the cost cutting. With Congress now examining Medicare's $16 billion annual doctor bill, the private sector will surely follow suit again.

Medicare's approach to hospital costs since 1983 has been to pay a set fee for each illness instead of paying whatever the hospital charges. If a hospital's costs are less than the reimbursement amount, the hospital keeps the difference. If the costs are greater, the hospital takes a hit.

But Washington's strategy for dealing with Medicare's ballooning tab from doctors is much different. The thrust of the proposed system is to make sure Medicare payments to specialists are related to the difficulty, stress, time and expense of the work. The plan being developed for Congress by the Harvard University School of Public Health for $2.5

million could cause dramatic drops in payments for certain types of surgery and boosts for diagnostic treatment.

Paying doctors according to the effort and cost of treatment makes sense—but may cause problems. Private insurance companies worry that lower Medicare payments for some services will push uncovered costs onto privately insured patients. Nor would the new payment scheme address directly the increased number of visits to doctors that have helped drive physician costs up 14 percent a year—triple the general inflation rate. When Congress considers a new scheme for doctor fees, it should continue to push for additional ways to bring the cost of the entire health system under control.

In the last decade, medical practice has changed drastically. Not the least of the changes is the manner in which doctors are compensated. The traditional fee-for-service system has well rewarded those physicians who do more, underscoring the principle that the more you do the more you get paid. Those who perform medical-surgical procedures are paid disproportionately more. Only recently has the issue been raised about whether the procedure or study is appropriate. It has, for example, been documented that one of the real risks associated with coronary artery bypass surgery is the possibility that the patient will have a stroke. Yet 14 percent of these bypass procedures recently were said by cardiologists reviewing the data to be unequivocally inappropriate.

One is compelled to ask such searching questions as: Why did the family doctor allow his patient to have that surgery? Was the doctor intimidated by the cardiac specialist? Does he play golf with that specialist? Or does he have a financial interest in the cardiac special studies unit with the cardiologist and thus prefers not to make waves? Or, in fact, is he just not able to make that kind of decision due to the limits of his knowledge? Who, then, will protect the patient?

In general, it is estimated that between 20 and 40 percent of procedures performed on patients aren't warranted. Needless to say, these procedures involve significant expenditures and the potential for serious problems caused by treatment and diagnosis

(called iatrogenesis). The physician in managed care is often willing to do the electrocardiogram (EKG) prior to sending the patient
to the cardiologist. But even though that specialist is sent the EKG,
he often deems it necessary to do his own on a similar machine.

The primary physician, in his role as a cost-efficient provider, is
thus placed in the position of deciding whether to call the cardiologist and ask him why he had to do another EKG. It has been shown
that there are 50 percent more EKGs and 40 percent more X-rays
done in fee-for-service medicine than in managed care. When
analyzed for appropriateness, these extra procedures or studies do
not appear necessary. But if not for medical necessity, then for
what? The cardiologist who does an echocardiogram in his office
as part of a routine exam and charges $400 to $500 for this defends
it on the basis of quality care. Yet it is difficult to discover where
the elements of quality are buried. For the truly honest physician,
a dilemma naturally arises as to whether he should do the procedure because he is engendering profit from it or because the
patient really needs it.

Likewise, it has been reported that from 25 to 40 percent of
hospitalizations are unnecessary. Several studies have shown that
managed care can reduce hospital costs 25 to 40 percent over the
traditional system without any alteration in the quality of care.
Medicine defends itself by supporting more as better quality.
Though we are all very much aware of the possible serious con-
sequences of being hospitalized, there are large numbers of unnecessary hospitalizations. Physicians must often measure the
appropriateness of care against their concern about the medical-
legal ramifications or their loyalty to "support" the hospital by
admitting their patients. The hospital may have bought the practice
and provided it with a staff or with equipment and financing.

Hospitals, in other words, are literally buying practices in order
to assure a constant flow of patients from these doctors. Perhaps
some of these patients could be treated and cared for in a less
costly, less intensive setting equally well. If the doctor has an
obligation to admit the patient but has lost his ability to make

appropriate judgments, he places all medicine in a precarious position. This problem is compounded by the hospital's "control" of the physician.

Should the physician be an advocate for the patient no matter what the cost? Is society willing to pay for "everything," or must the physician make certain decisions to limit inappropriate care? Does the fifty-seven-year-old woman need to see the dermatologist for her wrinkles because she demands it? Or does the physician's responsibility go deeper and relate to the necessity and obligation to provide this kind of care? If a third party refuses to allow a particular procedure or referral, the doctor faces the dilemma of getting everything done no matter the costs.

The problem raises some complexities. There are, for example, extraordinary demographic variations in the frequency of procedures. If you live in La Jolla, for example, we are told that you are three times as likely to have a coronary artery bypass procedure than if you are a resident of Palo Alto. In some areas, there is a twentyfold difference in the variation of such bypass procedures. So who bears the responsibility of restricting this type of procedure?

Also, the use of inappropriate prescriptions is a serious problem. Certainly, the incorrect prescribing, the mistakes, the use of dangerous combinations of medications, and the fraudulent misuse of the prescription insurance card all put the physician in a posture of increased risk. When a patient asks his physician to write a prescription in the name of the person who holds the prescription card instead of the noninsured patient, he places both physician and pharmacist in ethical and legal jeopardy.

Many specialists risk a reduction in their income if the findings of a Harvard study (reported by Martin Tolchin in the *New York Times,* September 29, 1988) become the criteria for payment to physicians. Will this further exacerbate the dilemma?

Washington—A major overhaul of Medicare payments to doctors in which some specialists would lose up to 50 percent of their Medicare revenue was recommended in a study ordered by Congress and commissioned by the Department of Health and Human Services.

The study, by the Harvard School of Public Health, created a new way of comparing medical specialties by setting up a "relative value scale." It would compensate doctors on the basis of the work they performed and the costs of their training and practices. The work components include the time spent on a procedure, the technical skills needed and the mental effort, judgment and stress involved.

On that basis, the study found that doctors had been overcompensated for "invasive" procedures like surgery and diagnostic tests compared with what they received for "cognitive" services, like office visits. As a result, heart surgeons and ophthalmologists would lose 40 to 50 percent of their Medicare revenues if the study's scale were implemented, while the payments to family practitioners would increase 60 to 70 percent.

The study endorses the view of critics who argue that doctors who offer services like office visits are not as well compensated for their time as those who perform surgery and expensive tests. A result, these critics say, is that some doctors will carry out more tests and operations than are medically necessary, adding to the overall cost of health care.

The media's glorification of new technology has created the perception that patients need and/or are entitled to all the new technology. The primary doctor must grapple with the decision of when to use the new technology and how frequently. But what is appropriate, and how can he deny access? In this age of malpractice, the physician is naturally insecure and does not want to take a wrong position in this difficult medical decision-making, especially with the demanding patient.

The medical-legal climate, of course, has affected the way doctors behave. One in every eleven physicians now is sued each year. Good communications skills and their use in the proper situation can forestall or entirely avoid litigation. What should we make of the much discussed "cost" of malpractice to the system? Although the actual premium is approximately 4 to 5 percent of the gross income of all physicians, the true expenditure for the health care system is estimated to be many billions of dollars. The physician faced with the patient who has only a minor injury, such as a sprain, now must face the likelihood of being sued if there is a minor fracture and the patient was not X-rayed. The case of practicing "defensive medicine" prevails because the X-ray turns out to be the solution. Faced with this great problem and the cost of care, it's obvious that physicians must rethink and redefine their decision-making process.

At the same time, with the advent of risk sharing in managed-care systems, the decisions physicians make about referrals and testing are likely to be affected by their concern over cost-effectiveness. If the decisions are made appropriately, this will enhance the delivery of medical care. Conversely, if these decisions are made inappropriately, medical care may be adversely affected. So the physician is faced by yet another obvious dilemma—is his decision cost-effective *and* appropriate?

Occasionally, too, a predicament is associated with a terminally ill patient. To balance between the law and the principle of "humanity to man," the wisdom of a King Solomon is required. The issue of euthanasia presents the doctor with the ultimate dilemma. Who has the right to decide, and is there ever a time when it is appropriate for a physician to actively participate in euthanasia?

As the issues become more complex, practicing physicians must face dilemmas such as these on a daily basis. Because they apply both individually and impact society's standards, each must be dealt with in an appropriate fashion in order to preserve the integrity, not to mention the cost-effectiveness, of medicine.

CHAPTER ◆ SIX

The Profit-versus-Nonprofit Myth

What are some of America's most widely accepted myths? Our country's leaders, though well intentioned, exhibit a great degree of naiveté, both personally and in their dealings with community problems. Their belief in nonprofit organizations linked to government support can solve our health care problems.

On an individual level, they hope to stop smoking before it hurts them. They take no precautions against AIDS because they think they're the lucky ones. Going through life, they may neglect health and/or financial security. They hope the problem of 3 million homeless Americans, whom they see every day on the way to work or shopping, will somehow solve itself.

On a national level, they believe that adverse federal economic conditions—whether regarding the national deficit, the trade imbalance, adequate defense needs, or foreign policy relations—will improve before the problems are really felt. Their premise is, of course, that the United States is a self-correcting society and that in a democracy the built-in constitutional check-and-balance system will prevail.

There is some element of truth in the idea that our system is self-correcting, but only when the problems are brought to light, probed deeply, and the vital need for a healing process is exposed. Then—and only then—does our highly valued check-and-balance mechanism function.

No myth is more pervasive, perhaps, than the belief that our national medical care system is necessarily wasteful because of our national wealth and immense resources. And within that myth is another—that nonprofit health institutions are really that. This attitude, in turn, fosters the initial premise that our medical institutions, as humane entities, are expensive, even exorbitant, because they have to be—"they help people."

But the truth is that nowhere in American society is there greater contradiction and greater hypocrisy than in the "not-for-profit" or nonprofit structure within our country's medical care delivery system. Hospitals, prepaid insurance programs, insurance companies, religious organizations, and other groups such as the Internal Revenue Service give tax breaks to these so-called nonprofit health care organizations, the 501C organizations that try so vigorously and so virtuously to gain tax-exempt benefits.

The nonprofit shield allows organizations to accept charitable donations, not pay taxes, and lobby for preferential legislation to encompass and protect their nonprofit status. Most of these nonprofit organizations maximize the reimbursement for hospital services and premium costs as much as for-profit organizations. An executive or other individual can easily make a career transition to a nonprofit hospital because it operates under the same protection and with the same philosophy as other business enterprises in the United States. And Blue Cross and Blue Shield are no exception. They, too, operate with the protection of nonprofitability but hold the same philosophies as for-profit insurance companies. The difference is, of course, that Blue Shield has physicians and Blue Cross has hospitals as its constituency.

Many of these nonprofit groups are blatant in their holier-than-thou behavior. They tell the public and insist to critics that they operate at a higher level of efficiency, with lower costs than their for-profit counterparts.

Yet, in practice, it's hard to tell the difference between the not-for-profit and the for-profit organizations. The nonprofit hospitals and other nonprofit groups turn to tax-free bonds and charitable fund-raising. They compete with the sale of stock or investing in risk capital or bonds that are available to the for-profit sector of the economy. The bonds sold for nonprofit hospitals, while usually tax-exempt, may not obtain the same degree of serious scrutiny as that given to securities issued for for-profit organizations. Perhaps the reason is that the philosophy of many investors is "Who ever heard of a hospital going out of business?" But they do, they certainly do. Those who buy such bonds will need more luck and a more realistic attitude if they aren't to lose their investment.

What further compounds the hypocrisy is that these nonprofit organizations build hospitals that have billing practices using max-imizers (which allow nonprofit hospitals to bill the maximum amounts) and operate with the same philosophy as for-profit hospitals that segregate money-making departments. So the nonprofit hospitals are also found segregating anesthesiology, radiology, and cardiology in a manner almost identical to that in the for-profit hospital setting.

As mentioned earlier, hospitals were built with the goal of serving the needs of humanity. In the various types of community, public, private, and specialized hospitals that developed over the years, the general concept of healing the ill remained, at least superficially, the objective. Obviously, nonprofit hospitals and other nonprofit organizations initially adopted the philosophy of charitable organizations serving the poor. In fact, charitable and religious orders became enthusiastic sponsors of nonprofit hospitals.

But it would be unrealistic and foolish for us to adhere to the historical concept that charitable health practice is still prevalent in our society. One cannot overlook the obvious fact that the not-for-profit hospitals have evolved into for-profit hospital chains or complexes, and nonprofit HMOs and Blue Cross plans involved in the American mainstream behave as any other for-profit ventures do.

It might be worthwhile at this point to offer a current medical-cost fact sheet to show why we need to erase the not-for-profit myth in our system:

◆ The not-for-profit institution spends more money that is not taxed and is able to maintain nonprofit status, while operating in other segments as a profit-making business. This practice contributes to what Robert H. Brook of the Rand Corporation estimates as the one-fifth of U.S. medical care that is unnecessary and wasteful. Either through taxation or private funding, this is costing the nation $120 billion a year.

◆ In many cases, this unneeded care is a result of financial incentives on the part of hospitals and doctors. But far more often it stems from inadequately informed physicians who do not realize that it will not help their patients.

Demonstrating its concern about quality issues, Congress passed a law calling on the Institute of Medicine of the National Academy of Sciences to design a strategy for processing and assuring the quality of care in the Medicare program.

◆ Edward J. Stemmler, the retired executive vice president of the University of Pennsylvania Medical Center, declared that he no longer has the kind of academic freedom to say, "I'm going to do it my way." Instead, he said, "There is a body of knowledge showing that there is a preferred way and I better damn well do it the preferred way." Medicine today has accepted preferred-treatment patterns.

◆ Robert J. Blendon, of the Harvard Medical School, said that 37 million Americans have no medical insurance and 13.5 million of them go without such crucial care as treatment of high blood pressure and diabetes because they can't afford it.

♦ The federal Health Care and Financing Administration surveyed the medical charts of hospital patients across the country and announced that more than 6 percent of all Medicare patients— that means almost 500,000 people—are receiving substandard care, whether too little or too much care.

♦ Allan M. Greenspan, a cardiologist specializing in electrophysiology at Albert Einstein Medical Center in Philadelphia, headed a team that reviewed the charts of Medicare patients who received cardiac pacemakers at local hospitals. Afterward, he concluded that 20 percent of the implants were inappropriate.

♦ After reviewing coronary artery bypass operations in three hospitals with a panel of experts, the Rand Corporation's Robert Brook concluded that the surgery was inappropriate or questionable in 44 percent of the cases. In another study, Brook found that more than 30 percent of patients who underwent carotid endarterectomy, a risky procedure to clear obstructions from arteries leading to the brain, did not need the operation.

These cases are not quoted here to prove that nonprofit health organizations that are actually for-profit create these problems. But they contribute to them by their unduly high costs and wrong emphasis. They are, in my opinion, one of the major sources of the problem. Their conduct mirrors their for-profit brethren.

Most nonprofit health organizations have a director or directress for the sole purpose of raising funds under the guise of a not-for-profit institution. This effort sometimes involves hiring for-profit organizations, at fees of several hundred thousand dollars, to raise several million dollars. This fund-raising may involve a capital fund-raising or new building program, a new equipment program, or some other type of program that the nonprofit administration decides is necessary for its growth at any particular time. Some of the more subtle ways of raising money are dances, cake sales, antique automobile sales, and a whole variety of other bazaars and funding vehicles using volunteers who freely provide their services and expertise. When these nonprofit operators hire consultants to help them maximize opportunities, we see the results in self-aggrandizing advertisements, proclamations of contributions, and the naming of facilities after contributors or celebrated patients. In visiting their facilities, it is not uncommon to see buildings and pavilions bearing the name of these benefactors or even to find rooms, chapels, water fountains, benches, chairs, elevators, libraries, and administrative offices also bearing those names. All the techniques of for-profit enterprise are enthusiastically applied to the not-for-profit groups, who still keep insisting that they are what they aren't.

As mentioned in an earlier chapter, perhaps the most hypocritical aspect of all is the creation by those nonprofit institutions of for-profit subsidiaries. The goal, of course, is to find further ways of maximizing cash flow for the parent organization. Some of these profit-making subsidiaries include real estate companies, service units such as laundry, food services, pharmacies, durable medical equipment, billing services, home care, management aid, and so on. In addition, the salaries of individuals paid to run the not-for-profit parent and those subsidiaries compare very favorably to those paid to the people in comparable-sized organizations in the for-profit sector.

Many of these nonprofit groups indulge in activities such as forming national organizations to help the group lobby and market their services and compete nationally. They, in turn, will also form allegiances with for-profit organizations if they meet both their marketing and lobbying objectives. Voluntary Hospitals of America, for example, has a coventure with Aetna Life and Casualty Company, a program called Partners. And many religious orders operate chains of hospitals with the same competitive zeal as their for-profit rivals.

In challenging the not-for-profit myth, I want to emphasize that I am certainly not opposed to charitable activities. I contribute heavily to many nonprofit organizations, such as the National Cancer Institute and various universities and geriatric centers. But I sometimes have to question the modus vivendi and behavior of the professional staffs that operate some of these facilities.

To take a holier-than-thou attitude but secretly and even openly compete in the profit arena while maintaining a tax-free stance is wrong. Not only does the contradiction in attitude and conduct confuse the organization's mission, but it results in runaway waste in our health system and totally fools the public or anyone else who is unaware of the real facts. If one's mission is to serve the poor and needy, this philosophy should be supported and protected by society—as long as the mission is legitimate. All civilized societies have the responsibility of caring for the needy. But it is foolish and wasteful to allow our health care system to suffer the lie of nonprofit when the profit motive lies just under the surface.

In short, charitable endeavors should be charitable and the mission of these institutions should be to serve the needy. But more than a few nonprofit hospitals have been known to turn away the sick and needy for lack of proper insurance coverage. And when the public reads about this type of abuse, it is understandably horrified and confused—and then quickly forgets.

The myth needs to be overhauled. If hospitals conduct themselves as for-profit businesses, they should be taxed as everyone else is and not given preferential treatment.

CHAPTER ◆ SEVEN

An International
Health Care Scoreboard

Americans, the world's big spenders on health care, do not receive the greatest benefits from their system. Other countries that spend a lesser portion of their gross national product on it provide health care for their citizens that is at least equal to and often better than ours.

At the same time, almost every other country has problems in their health delivery systems, including cost overruns and organizational foul-ups. But I think it is possible for us to learn from both their advantages and their difficulties. For the purpose of an international comparison, we will discuss the countries that Americans most often associate with in sizing up our relative performance. They are the United Kingdom, Canada, West Germany, Italy, France, Switzerland, Japan, Israel, and the South American countries.

Let us compare the systems of health care in Great Britain and Canada. In the United Kingdom, under the National Health Service (NHS), the government owns the facilities and employs the doctors. The differences in the Canadian system are that the federal government and the provincial governments join in providing the financial resources for a tax-supported insurance system in which the hospital payments are fixed. The ten Canadian provinces negotiate annual budgets with each province's hospital and medical associations. This places a cap on the total cost of health care expenditures. The individual association then places an allotment for fees for physicians. Physicians are paid out of the provinces' funds, and are strictly forbidden to bill patients, an exception being for some types of equipment.

In the United Kingdom, the NHS pays family practitioners an annual amount for each patient, similar to a capitation. Great Britain, unlike Canada, does allow physicians to practice outside the system. Budget restrictions in both countries have been responsible for delays in care up to six months. In the English system, the infrastructure is crumbling compared to a stronger hospital network in Canada.

Another example is Cuba, which recently opened its doors to the American media in an attempt to reattract tourists. And along with that, the Cubans are permitting the world to share an interesting turnaround in their health care experience. Their primary care results are being credited by them for longer life expectancy, from a low of fifty years some thirty years ago to a high of seventy years at the present time. Also interesting is their disclosure that they are selling high-tech surgery such as open-heart procedures and organ transplants to the South American countries. While I do not fully accept what must at least in part be propaganda by Fidel Castro, the head of state, even if we believe only a portion of the claims, the Cubans' case for primary care in underdeveloped countries is probably well founded.

What can we draw from that? Medical reform can be structured in most countries when a commonsense approach to health care is adopted. High tech is not the answer when only a very small percentage of individuals need procedures such as nuclear medicine, CAT scans, magnetic resonance imaging, lithotripsy, and transplants; but the majority of people will benefit from a soundly developed primary care program when easily accessible concerned physicians can guide health care needs.

In Japan the extraordinary length of the average hospital stay, which is triple ours, as well as the alarming incidence of cancer, will inevitably lead the Japanese to reassess their future health care needs. They will probably look to some manner of managed health care program that will allow them to deliver health care at lower cost.

In many ways, we can benefit from studying what evolves in Japan because that country's great technological skills and its people's work ethic could offer an example, or even a role model, for us. The fact that the Japanese economy is soaring while also creating great future problems has a direct relevance to our country and that, too, should compel us to watch the evolution of their health care process. This crowded country will recognize economic opportunity in managed health care.

Other countries, too, offer relevant problems. In Oslo, Norway, recent newspaper headlines of a child whose arm was broken and who was shuttled around for half a day because the injury occurred outside her family's provided health care sector are something that is not unfamiliar to us.

In Great Britain, the long queues that are typically part of that nation's health care system are evidence that a new approach is badly needed there as it is, indeed, in the world at large. Our system is hardly so sound that we can be smug or self-satisfied. Later in this chapter, I will discuss the U.K. system in much greater detail. But at this juncture it should be noted that even in a cursory look at the United Kingdom, it is clear that amid the crushing national deficit the National Health Service faces a crisis in funds and innumerable delays.

In Sweden, often cited as a model of social welfare, equality of opportunity and benefits is tinged with inefficiency. Obviously, new incentives are needed to gain greater efficiency. Incentives should be created for managed health care, management improvement, and better vital data.

Around the world, especially in the Far East, health care is becoming a major concern for industrial management in such countries as Taiwan, Malaysia, Indonesia, and Singapore. In the Mideast, the same problems exist. There are massive difficulties, and such international bodies as the United Nations International Development Association, the Asian Development Group, and the World Bank are grappling with them to provide help.

In Israel health care is delivered by an organization known as Kopat Holime, operating within the context of a socialist system. Emerging in a pioneering country that needed to treat many individuals suffering from malaria, as well as many serious medical problems for the thousands of Holocaust survivors, this managed health care system now finds itself under tremendous pressure due to overutilization and improper financing. The Israeli government is stymied in its efforts to provide additional services, partly because its health care system was initially developed on the basis of low-cost, controlled services.

Students of health care systems have a particular fascination for the English system. Let's take a more comprehensive look at the national health care system in the United Kingdom, which has been both praised and criticized and is often studied as a worldwide role model.

For a variety of reasons, including its privatization component, the U.K. health care system presents a new area of opportunity for managed health care. The government is seeking an evaluation of alternatives and is attempting to find new ways to collect data. And, despite its privatization, there appears to be a growing sentiment for a shift to a public-private partnership in managed health care. The National Health Service is looking for ways to jointly finance same-day surgery units for the private sector.

On its own, the private system is active. The private insurance companies finance private hospital wings and buy national health insurance with support services. Private hospitals buy land from the National Health System to construct new facilities that will share support services. The private sector is also buying underutilized facilities such as those for breast cancer screening and infertility services. There are ventures to jointly finance magnetic-resonance-imaging centers and lithotripsy equipment. Private companies are recognizing a need in the British health care system and are forming private ventures to establish for-profit entities to provide these services. This infrastructure of the British system needs this private initiative; currently, the Thatcherites are attempting to pave the way for this type of activity.

As they study the public and private sectors with an entrepreneurial eye, the managed health care companies will certainly consider voucher systems and a type of voucher system for supplemental services will become part of the total delivery system. It is safe to say that there is both the demand and the motivation to provide a supplementary service to the NHS network.

But the process in the United Kingdom of adopting sensible changes in its system is arousing critics as well as adherents. Two groups have taken a similar approach. The Institute of Economic Affairs, recognized as a body prone to support Prime Minister Margaret Thatcher, sided with the Centre for Policy Studies, which declared, "It is not possible to simply adopt an American model." Nonetheless, the Centre felt that HMOs offered important lessons for Great Britain. The only difference between the two groups' positions was the IEA's contention that consumers should register with a general practitioner who would then affiliate with a health management unit, or HMU, rather than choose an American-style HMO.

Adding to the debate, the *Financial Times* noted that the operation of HMOs in the United States depends upon diverse market suppliers. In America there is a surplus of hospitals and physicians in most metropolitan areas with large populations, which allows for negotiation for better rates. In Britain most people depend on a large, local hospital in their district. Hence, the newspaper concluded, the new HMOs would cause people to travel large distances and as a result choice and competition would be reduced.

No doubt fueling the debate was the formation in 1984 of a form of HMO introduced into the National Health Service called the

IMA, or more formally, the Independent Medical Associates. This IMA operates the private Harrow Health Care Center in London.

The debate included the Conservative Research Department characteristically asserting, "More radical ideas such as reform of GPOs into HMOs are unlikely to be adopted." Another group apparently fearing for its existence, the National Association of Health Authorities, attacked proposals to replace health authorities with boards of commissioners. This, the organization charged, would stifle "innovative" approaches to health care.

And so the debate went on, not too different perhaps than that in the United States. Meanwhile, pressure groups continue to do their best to hammer out compromises furthering their own interests.

Less a subject of debate is the mutuality of concern that exists around the world on the need for better, more cost-effective health care. In 1988 foreign visitors studying HMOs came to this country from Great Britain, Japan, Sweden, Australia, Italy, and the Philippines. And the list of arrivals continues to increase as more international companies grow aware of the health care options and opportunities.

Among the American companies offering HMO opportunities to foreign companies are U.S. Healthcare, Cigna Corporation, Aetna Life & Casualty Insurance, and American International Healthcare, as well as consulting groups such as Birch and Davis. In Great Britain, the United States is represented by such hospital management companies as American Medical International, Hospital Corporation of America, and National Medical Enterprises.

As in our country, there is a sizeable waste in foreign medical delivery systems. And there are also large variations in medical procedures, hospital utilization, and related charges and costs. Most foreign countries do not have an excess of hospital beds. They did not follow our example of enacting a Hill-Burton law that was then Medicare-linked to a tax-spending spree to fund new hospitals. Further, most countries outside the United States do not embrace practices in which groups of physicians form a single medical delivery unit and any attempt to start them has been vigorously opposed, especially in Germany.

Around the world, there is, however, a large indemnity insurance market in place. The programs are largely composed of hospitals and physicians practicing American-style medicine, but they, too, are facing similar problems. Most of these foreign health insurance organizations and companies are suffering from overextended benefits in both the private and public sectors.

Obviously, as the new dawn of the Common Market arrives in 1992 and trade and cultural barriers are lowered on the European continent, there will be an international need for better management and greater sharing of health care resources.

Despite the many current problems, one cannot but feel that better things are ahead. I expect Japan to move into a better and more controlled health care market. I think Israel will lead the Mideast in reform to meet the crisis of undercapacity and increased demand in an economy strapped for resources. And I think that the Scandinavian countries are clearly moving to refine their government-supported health care systems. In the United Kingdom, the debate will lead to positive interaction between the private and public sectors. All in all, there is a great vacuum to be filled, and I sense great change coming and greater opportunity beckoning for well-focused innovation on a global basis.

Creating Marketplace Competition

Whether some care to admit it or not, competition and mass production are as crucial to our enterprise system as the brain-power and organic fuel that power it. Any skeptic need only look at how products such as automobiles, radios and television sets, computers, and homes have become accessible through mass pricing to millions after their introduction at astronomical prices. And quality has improved along with availability. This development can be seen in services of all kinds, with the exception of health care.

For years medical care remained the sole province of physicians and hospitals and their associates. So tight a grip did they have on this monopoly that patients often placed themselves in untenable circumstances. Even asking some probing questions about one's own body could bring a frown of displeasure.

Patients were not informed of their rights, let alone given a fair indication of what was really wrong with them or what was going to be done to their bodies. Because they were protected and insulated from normal marketplace forces, physicians and hospitals were able to wield tremendous amounts of power and influence.

Here and there, a natural competitive force began to enter the field. But even today in our so-called advanced, democratic society, many physicians like to argue that "things were better before marketplace forces started to influence the economics of health care."

Yet I, for one, believe that competition is an important, cost-effective health care component. Marketplace competition disseminates information and educates individuals about the outcome, costs, quality, and comparative reputations of health care institutions. The resulting concern about loss of market share has already led to a scramble in paid notices in the media as to how they are "unique" in their field. Unfortunately, because competition and advertising are relatively new to the health care marketplace, we are being subjected to exaggerated claims and hype that confuse consumers and would be difficult to substantiate if challenged.

So what do we read and observe on television? A giant, urban hospital complex tells us that it was responsible for the development of a new healing process. That it saved the lives of a stricken child or adult. That its services are available to the indigent as well as to the affluent. An intensifying race is on—as it is among makers of toothpaste, cars, and perfumes—for our attention as hospitals advertise, physicians advertise, HMOs advertise, nursing homes advertise. All are striving to capture our attention and a greater share of the health care dollar. Indeed, hospitals today are employing advertising and public relations agencies and have set up their own internal advertising capabilities to devote $1 million or more a year to media advertising and exposure.

Seeking to enhance their competitive position, hospitals also have installed "boutiques" that offer weight reduction, programs for eating disorders, cardiac rehabilitation, cosmetic surgery, gymnasiums, surgicenters, food and catering services, baby-sitting services for the very young and the elderly, plus a plethora of other marketable services.

But does all this hype, marketing flurry, and service segmentation really constitute competition? I don't think so.

As a devoted advocate of true capitalism and the power of the marketplace, I believe that in a real economic marketplace the parasitic stranglehold that hospital-based physicians have on their "host" hospitals must and can be broken. The fact is that radiologists, anesthesiologists, and other providers of health care services want to remain immune from competitive forces in the marketplace.

Our company's hospital negotiators can relate numerous examples of a hospital being unable to arrive at a reasonable contract that is beneficial to the economic health of the institution because the hospital-based physicians want to be paid full fee-for-service, regardless of what others in the marketplace ask for similar services. This double billing grew out of the Medicare mentality of maximizing reimbursement. Radiologists bill for the technical component, or use of the equipment, as one bill, and have a separate fee for interpretation. This type of billing methodology is employed by many hospital-based physicians in other specialties such as cardiology and neurology. Thus, in effect, hospitals have created Frankenstein monsters that hold them captive to a billing mechanism that is no longer relevant in a powerful, competitive health care environment.

Marketplace forces and the creation of marketplace competition provide a broader variety of health care products and services and directly affect their cost, but they also push providers into revealing who they really are. This rivalry has unearthed some rather nasty behavior in the provider community. Hospitals in Pittsburgh have banded together to keep competition out and maintain the status quo. In other cities around the country, physicians and dentists have joined to fix prices and avoid competition. Recently, the Justice Department inaugurated an investigation and it was proceeding at this writing.

Inevitably, as marketplace forces pervade, we will surely witness more of these abuses and illegal acts, as well as evidence of unnecessary services. Several newspapers have recently cited studies disclosing the unwarranted number of caesarian sections performed on pregnant women. This is only one example of the 20 percent of U.S. health care that is unnecessary. I believe that the marketplace will further unearth unneeded medical practices. But as competition increases within the provider community and the selection of providers and services becomes increasingly based on economic and marketplace consideration, I think that unnecessary medical procedures will decline.

What will bring about more marketplace competition? It will inevitably flow from the exorbitantly high cost of services and the growing scrutiny that these are arousing. But I am enough of a realist to know that true competition can only develop from enlightenment in the medical community, federal and local governments, and a greater awareness on the part of the public regarding the need for a freer health care marketplace.

As these changes occur, I see the following advantages of marketplace competition:

◆ Scrutiny of comparative services will demonstrate the positive or negative aspects of individual providers in our system.

◆ Economic pressure on services will make them more cost-effective.

◆ Marketplace pressure will improve quality of services.

◆ As curiosity about costs creates a need for information, the confusion and mystery surrounding many medical procedures, or at least some of their intricacies, will be clarified.

◆ A better-educated patient and public will permit a better choice of physician and hospital.

◆ We will get a better value for our health care dollar.

◆ Health care will become susceptible to the forces of supply and demand. This has not yet been the case. But when it does, price or costs will inevitably respond to the greater volume of use.

Today, however, in such areas as CAT scans, lithotriptors, and other high-tech procedures, price increases with popularity because this technology so far is restricted by the number of health institutions that have them available.

♦ Large-scale purchasers of health care such as third-party insurance companies and HMOs will be held accountable and in turn will hold their providers accountable. An example of this is the purchasing of laboratory services from one national company and the ability to negotiate quality and cost. This has created a dramatic reduction in the cost of such things as laboratory procedures, mental health services, radiology services, podiatry services, durable medical equipment, and the appropriate use of various hospital services.

♦ Consumers will no longer buy Blue Cross or indemnity insurance products without shopping around. And the competition in the marketplace will allow individuals to be educated as to the benefits of various products. As they learn more about the service quotient and quality of various products, consumers no longer will merely choose a product or service because it has had a monopoly in the marketplace. The oligopoly of the Blue Cross plans and large insurance companies will crumble under the forces of marketplace competition.

What will all this lead to? A higher-quality, more efficient, and more cost-effective health care system, certainly a goal that all of us want to reach.

CHAPTER ◆ NINE

The Boons of a Monitoring System

If anyone still doubts the urgent need to bring our medical costs down, consider the following:

Aetna Life and Casualty Company has asked its customers to report doctors they suspect of insurance fraud. After conducting a 700-household survey, the big insurer decided to enlist the public in its offensive against runaway health care costs. Four out of every ten consumer respondents said they believe that their doctors have cheated an insurance company at least one time.

The Congressional Budget Office estimated that federal spending on health would grow 20 percent between 1987 and 1989, exceeding increases for other major federal budget items. For example, military spending was expected to increase 5.7 percent, Social Security spending 12.4 percent, and interest on the national debt 17.8 percent.

How much, percentage-wise, is Uncle Sam paying of the total health bill? In 1987 government paid 41 percent of it, private insurers paid 34 percent, and individual patients 25 percent, according to the Health Care Financing Administration. But as the *New York Times* reported in November 1988, the federal government and private insurers were able to control hospital costs by setting ceilings on the fees paid for hospital care of various illnesses. Still, overall costs continued to soar in spite of intermittent government attempts to freeze physician fees and to restrain doctors from charging patients more than Medicare allows.

Unfortunately, most corporate executives view health care costs as a matter of major concern only about once a year. That is when the chief financial officer reports that the company's health care costs have jumped once again, anywhere from 20 to 50 percent over the year before. The CFO then notifies the chief executive officer that the company has only two options—either to absorb the extra costs by cutting into its bottom line or by effecting a cost shift to the employees.

The latter, of course, is an especially delicate business. Most CFO's usually approach this step by asking their benefits officer or insurance consultant to try to find new ways to reduce benefits without creating too much of a stir among the company's employees. This is obviously a shortsighted solution. It will not work because health care costs continue to escalate. It is my estimate that most companies are realizing year-to-year cost rises between 20 and 40 percent for their 1989 budgets and many are higher. Increases will continue well into the 90s. Thus, when one cost shifts and places an increased burden on the employee, it is in essence forcing a salary decrease on the employee. And it goes without saying that in today's competitive marketplace, this salary decrease could easily work against keeping valuable employees. How many companies can afford that?

Meanwhile, in an effort to ferret out new ways of controlling their health care costs, companies today are purchasing software reporting systems that will tell their key executives exactly how medical services are actually spent for the benefits being purchased. I endorse this effort of trying to hold the provider community accountable. It is certainly a positive step toward having the company involve itself more in a corrective program attacking the ever increasing cost of doing business. But it is not enough. We must use this information derived through sophisticated technology to negotiate better value for our health care dollar, to get more out of better provider contracts.

The trend toward holding our hospitals, physicians, and ancillary medical delivery components accountable for their costs is a very strong step in the right direction for American industry.

Until now most purchasers and recipients of health care have been insulated from the real bills. For companies that are self-insured (companies accept the full risks, and pay a third party for administration of claims), the insurance company merely pays the bills and pays full charges. The company executives do not see the actual bills. These charges are also increasing at an intensified rate as hospitals shift costs and charges away from Medicare and managed health care programs toward corporations and insurance companies and private pay patients paying a higher portion of health care costs. To explain: Many companies are being sold a bill of goods by third-party administrators and by insurance companies giving them this sort of sales pitch—"We'll process your paper and you will be self-insured. Therefore, by maintaining your cash flow, this will bring about a positive impact on your bottom line." This benefit is usually short-lived as more companies find that insurance companies charge more for processing more paper, and the more bills insurance companies and third-party administrators pay, the more paper they process. Some large companies, such as Prudential, are changing this policy after a decade of endorsing self-insurance.

In today's world, there's a hard fact in our health care system. Where Medicare is trying to limit increases to 3 to 4 percent and managed health care companies are working to negotiate better hospital and physician contracts, the hospitals are left to depend upon those who pay full charges. These are usually the indemnity companies and those companies that traditionally recognize full-charge bills from hospitals and physicians. Usually, it's the self-insured or ASO, the "administrative service only" insurance programs that generate a profit, not the insuring entity taking the full risk.

Now let's examine how we can best monitor health care costs and how these must take effect in major areas.

Hospital services must be comparative. In other words, we must be able to compare similar services with competitive hospitals in a specific area. When these reports are submitted, the employer will readily see that there is a great variance in fees from one hospital to another. Some will defend it. For example, the academic institutions will say, "Well, certainly there must be higher costs because we have to reflect the cost of education." This is a fallacy. Our medical school hospitals receive tuition and subsidies from governmental agencies. They also receive support from affluent members of the community and from foundations. Education must be segregated from other health care costs.

I have no argument with society supporting an educational effort to help our teaching hospitals. But I am concerned when costs are piled one on top of another. And when they finally reach the patient, these costs have been greatly expanded and even exaggerated. I recommend that both the services and their fees start with the actual services rendered to the patient and then be traced back to the direct, not the compounded, costs.

This process will give the purchaser a much clearer, more direct way of evaluating the actual against the inflated costs and a better understanding of what the true costs really are. As I have stated earlier, I believe that most hospitals today are building their accounting systems by optimizing and maximizing those systems. And in doing so, they are deluding themselves—and everyone else—into believing that the resulting costs are the real costs, which every year become part of their operating systems. One can only conclude that most hospitals do not know what their real costs are. They must if many are to survive.

Since the issue of financing teaching hospitals often arises, it might be worthwhile to consider them at this point.

Medical-school tuitions these days average $15,000 a year, but our medical schools claim that they can't possibly afford to educate doctors at those costs. They claim costs are between $40,000 and $50,000 a year. Furthermore, the salaries for interns and residents are certainly quite nominal compared to the effort that they put forth and the amount of hours that they work. Hospitals again explain that this is part of the cost of an education and an educational system. But I believe that these costs should be isolated from community medical care. The educational system should be considered one segment of our society and the delivery of health care should be another segment. Thereby, we would be able to readily appraise what these actual costs are.

Secondly, I believe that the community will certainly pay for health care which is above the norm or which reaches to the point of excellence. In a capitalistic society, it is axiomatic that there is always room for higher-priced service or products and there is also room for competitively priced service and products. As I have urged before, we must inject competition into the health care arena. The data reports that we referred to a bit earlier will actually allow executives to analyze the services they are purchasing in a competitive environment. And since we all pay taxes, it is certainly fair to assess our tax system for medical education.

If competition is the way of the marketplace, when hospital and physician bills reach the real payer, then a monitoring system of health care costs will come into play, exerting a positive effect on costs.

While I do not want to recommend one software package over another, I do want to encourage the following monitoring practices:

- ◆ Get copies of all medical expenses.

- ◆ Set up informed review procedures.

- ◆ Create a modus operandi, including negotiating with providers and contracting with a company that is prepared to negotiate for you.

◆ Don't take the risks unless you really have to. That's not your business.

◆ The chief executive officer and the chief financial officer should involve themselves in this important cost decision.

◆ CEO—remember that you set the policies for the entire company. Your benefits officers must and will take their lead from you.

The fact we must recognize is that all services and products in a competitive society need to be monitored. When output is reviewed, quality inevitably improves. Thus, the medical care community should be accountable in its costs to the users and payers of its services.

Additionally, monitoring techniques should definitely compare the following:

◆ Level of patient satisfaction

◆ Outcome results

◆ Treatment patterns

◆ Readmission statistics

◆ Infection rates

◆ Mortality

◆ Costs, both overall and individual

◆ Duration of treatment

◆ Comparison to empirical standards

◆ Peer review

◆ Unrelated complications

◆ Preventive treatment

Without question, educating the purchasing public will lead to objective recognition of standards for quality care. And the monitoring system with built-in, objective criteria will remove the substandard and often more costly medical providers from the marketplace. Talented, dedicated providers will surely be recognized and rewarded. I sincerely believe in incentives for those who do more and get better results.

If the monitoring systems are put into effect and become available for inspection, they will result in a tacit or perhaps a formal "seal of approval." Most people behave best when their work is graded and reviewed. Sound, cost-effective, quality medical care should be the standard in our health care system, not the exception.

By way of emphasis, I would like to repeat some of the remarks by Dr. Michael A. Stocker, senior vice president for the New York region of U.S. Healthcare, given in July 1988 on behalf of the American Medical Care and Review Association before the Physician Payment Review Commission in Washington, D.C.

He endorsed such methods as the monitoring of visit rates and hospitalization rates to detect underutilization; a systematic monitoring of all grievances and inquiries that would indicate if the services are inappropriately withheld; an examination of transfers and terminations from individual physician offices; and the review of medical records to see if they conform to the standards of medical care as determined by quality assurance committees run by physicians.

Discussing the policies of U.S. Healthcare in connection with those practices, Dr. Stocker said: "This information when brought together systematically can be reviewed monthly and individual physicians are formally recertified on an annual basis. A physician who has raised significant barriers to care is asked to leave the program. This review mechanism requires in our system the annual review of approximately fifty thousand individual medical records, individual visits by trained staff to every primary physician at least six times a year, and individual physician visits by a plan medical director to every primary care physician's office annually."

Dr. Stocker continued: "We have also established a program which is now eight months old that increases payment to physicians for better-quality care. Physicians who perform well on chart audits, transfer rates between offices, member satisfaction, and demonstrated proficiency in managed care receive additional money in our reimbursement system. As you are probably aware by now, this is consistent with our general philosophy that appropriate rewards for superior managed care are the best way to objectively improve quality of care, member satisfaction, and the utilization of services. There is no magic about a system of this kind. It simply requires application and a general willingness to go to the trouble of gathering this information, and the will to act on it appropriately. Based on our experience, we believe it is feasible to design quality assurance systems that adequately monitor physician incentives."

It might also be added that no professional worth his or her salt would or should object to a monitoring process.

Data collection is important only if it is analyzed by knowledgeable people, who in turn can take appropriate action. Some organizations collect all types of data, perform the analysis, but are unable to take action. My charge to industry leaders is to monitor the action phase of data collection and analysis. Make sure there is a real payoff to your data collection effort.

CHAPTER ◆ TEN

A Wake-up Call
for Business and
Government

For many years, corporations—industry leaders with otherwise aggressive business strategies—have had to settle for defensive tactics when managing health care costs. But it hasn't helped them much to cut their employee cost burden.

Similarly, the federal government has reacted to demands for help in financing health care by continuously opening its coffers. This, too, has hardly contributed to meeting the pragmatic need to control costs in the nation's health care system.

Why link business and government together to cope with our ever rising health care costs? And how can this be done in view of the mounting needs and the millions of Americans who are largely or entirely uncovered?

Linking them is sensible since, in many ways, they hold the answer to the entire national problem. Consumers do, too, of course, and we will discuss them in the next chapter.

Health care adds $600 to the price of every automobile produced by Chrysler Corporation, says Joseph Califano, Jr., a former secretary of health, education and welfare, who is now on Chrysler's board of directors. And during the first nine months of 1987, General Motors Corporation had profits of $2.7 billion but spent $2 billion on employee medical care, or a 30 percent increase over the prior year. Similar problems faced the Southern New England Telephone Company, when in 1987 the company spent close to $40 million on medical expenses, or 14 percent more than the year before and more than double the amount of five years earlier.

These companies are not alone. Businesses of all sizes are threatened by costs they do not know how to control. Often they are too busy to cope with them, but they ignore the financial benefits of cutting waste and unproductive health care outlays. Their problems, too, are often passed on to their employees through steep increases in payroll deductions. Obviously, the time has come for business to demand a team approach to health care cost control, which can only be managed through a partnership among providers, insurers, business, and employees; each of these "partners" has a role to play.

In business, management must learn to be tougher at negotiation, to harness the clout of the great number of employees for whom they provide medical coverage. This is not to say that some companies aren't taking positive, creative steps. Consider the Xerox Corporation, which plans to establish a selective nationwide managed-care network. Pleased with the results of the HMOs in which more than 40 percent of its 60,000 employees participate, Xerox hopes to redirect as many as 80 percent into even more selective managed-care programs. Allied-Signal, Southwestern Bell, and Quaker Oats are already providing incentives for their employees to operate within such a managed health care program. And many smaller companies are beginning to band together with managed-care companies to achieve similar savings.

With a little creative initiative, a great deal can be done. Some employers are offering economic incentives if their employees use managed-care networks and are more aggressive about preventive care measures; companies such as Allied-Signal reward their employees who use a closed system rather than the open fee-for-service one with expanded medical benefits.

As stated before, the national cost of American health care is now about $600 billion a year. Our percent of GNP expenditures for it exceeds those of almost every other country—more than double that of France, West Germany, Japan, the Netherlands, or the United Kingdom. And with such a burden, we must be concerned that those costs do not contribute to making us a second-class economy. As a society, we have the responsibility to look upon health care as one of the resources, but not the only one, necessary to sustain a healthy, growing democratic environment. We must, in other words, learn to trade off one need for another but in the process ensure that the varying needs are fully met.

In addition, our federal government is wrestling with the problem of 37 million Americans who do not have adequate insurance or none at all, for whom the cost of providing sufficient insurance could reach between $15 and $30 billion per year depending upon the comprehensiveness of the health care package.

How much can the government afford, already paying as much as 41 percent of the national burden and with costs climbing seemingly without interruption? Despite recent efforts to control costs by setting ceilings for the treatment of various illnesses, there seems to be nothing that the federal government can do to keep costs down.

In our society, there are times when business and government have appeared to have an adversarial relationship, but there are other times—during wars or national emergencies, for example—when their ability to act together has sparked both admiration and significant results. I believe that the only way that business and government can meet this national emergency is to link arms to solve the current health care crisis. But first they, and we, must fully understand why these costs are increasing each year. To do so, let's examine some of the issues that are not apparently available to the public.

In some states, such as New York and New Jersey, there are

hospital rate-setting commissions. These commissions are highly influenced by the lobbying activities of the hospital community, which has demonstrated an insatiable appetite for yearly fee increases.

As mentioned earlier, rather than working toward greater efficiency, hospital managements are adding marketing departments and additional layers of administration. They seem to be more concerned about maintaining their position in the marketplace, when they should recognize that society has the right to receive health care that is competitive and is marketplace-driven and that both government and business would benefit from it. It helps no one, least of all those hospitals, to employ Madison Avenue advertising and public relations agencies to present an aura of medical glamour.

In 1989 both New York and New Jersey realized increased hospital costs of about 30 percent. But one can hardly accept this rise as final or warranted since, based on recent experience, the hospital community will soon ask for more. Such rises could be substantially reduced if efficiency became a high priority on the hospitals' list of objectives.

Even within that ever-rising cost syndrome, there is a new wrinkle, raising some troubling questions. This development involves the hospitals' sale of their facilities back to their physicians, making them partners not only in their ownership but in the process of maintaining high costs. The ramifications of this practice to business and government are hardly to be ignored because it appears to build a firmer springboard for rising health care costs.

Furthermore, we are seeing in our country as part of a coalition between government and business a move toward a form of national health insurance. This will supposedly give all Americans guaranteed access to health services. It is being called "universal health care." It first appeared prominently in Massachusetts when Governor Michael Dukakis created a universal health care program. It was then projected nationally during the presidential campaign when Governor Dukakis extolled its virtues as the Democratic candidate in 1988.

More recently, three new plans for revamping the existing system of health coverage have been proposed by economists and health authorities. Early in 1989, a broad coalition of government, industry, and health care sources called for a system in which all Americans would be covered for a basic package of medical services financed by private and governmental agencies. Supporting the new program, Professor Uwe Reinhardt, an economics professor at Princeton University and a member of the National Leadership Commission on Health Care, as the coalition was called, declared that the reason for the new program was "wholesale dissatisfaction with the current system." And Dr. John R. Ball, executive vice president of the American College of Physicians, said, "When you begin to see such a variety of groups all beginning to say the same basic thing, I think you begin to build a consensus."

So some experts back universal health coverage, supported by their recognition that the existing system is costly, wasteful, and full of gaps and inequities. Whether such a program will work remains to be seen, but first much more research is required not only on its implementation and operations but on how it will be financed. Will its sponsors be able to build into it cost-efficiencies that won't further burden both business and government?

The fact is that both government and business are locked into a state of helpless confusion because the former is afflicted with a horrendous deficit while the latter is frustrated by its inability to control those mounting health care costs. Despite numerous efforts to economize, health care spending grew about 5 percent a year between 1980 and 1986. Business currently picks up much of the $600 billion price tag for health care, but there's little doubt that both government and business will be forced to finance the proposed universal health care program if it becomes a reality.

Meanwhile, in January 1989 the Wyatt Company in Washington, D.C., estimated that the average cost of family medical care coverage would reach $3,000 per employee in 1989 if the health care inflation rate continued. In 1988 employer and employee contributions for family comprehensive medical care rose almost 12 percent to $2,700, compared with $2,412 the year before, Wyatt said. This means that medical care coverage exceeds 10 percent of compensation of many employees, Wyatt added.

In an interview in the January 1989 issue of *Business Insurance* magazine, Lance Tane, a consultant in Wyatt's New York office and chairman of Wyatt's group-flex practice, observed that in view of the enormous costs involved, employers should now rethink their benefit design plans. "Is the purpose of a medical plan to pay for ordinary expenses or is it only to pay for significant, unanticipated expenses that cause hardship?" he asked. "And if business believes it is the latter, then a closer, more strategic look at their plans is needed," he said.

The enormity of the $3,000 spent per employee is evident when contrasted with the amounts expended in other countries in 1989. In Canada the figure was slightly under $1,400 per person. In Switzerland and Sweden, it was about $1,200; in France and West Germany, about $1,000. And in Japan, it ranged between $800 and $900.

Consider other facts about the cost spiral. The cost of employer-sponsored health insurance plans rose an average 18.6 percent in 1988, according to Foster & Higgins, a national employee benefits firm. I believe that the cost will rise an equal amount in 1989. The Health Care Financing Administration, the agency that operates Medicare, estimates that spending will reach $1.5 trillion, or 15 percent of the country's entire economic output by the year 2000. And some investigators believe that Medicare spending eventually may outstrip the amount spent for Social Security benefits as the country enlarges its social welfare program.

In fact, it is the ever-increasing costs, as much as any other factor, which have caused business leaders to consider universal health coverage, says Dr. Stuart Altman, dean of the Brandeis University School of Public Health and a member of the national commission.

The broad-based coalition that has examined the universal

health program proposes to extend health coverage to the unin-sured by building on the current private-public health insurance system. But it stops short of recommending a government-controlled health system like that in Great Britain. Obviously, the coalition does not care to espouse a system sure to arouse great political controversy. Morris B. Abram, a lawyer and former chairman of the President's Commission for the Study of Ethics in Medicine, has admitted that it is a politicized issue. And Dr. Ball of the American College of Physicians, a consultant to the commis-sion, said, "It's important that it is pointed out that this universal health care is not socialized medicine."

In view of its importance, it is worth exploring the commission's thinking on the universal health proposal. Coalition members noted that there is a significant difference between a national system for financing health care coverage and a nationalized sys-tem for providing health care as in the British example. The coalition proposed keeping private health insurance in place by creating a separate fund known as the Universal Access Insurance Pool. But Professor Alain Enthoven, a respected health care econ-omist at Stanford University, who published his own proposal for universal health insurance, worried that in an era of budget-breaking deficits there will not be the political will to pursue universal health coverage.

Others were also worried that the entrenched institutions, such as the health insurance industry and the American Medical Asso-ciation, might oppose proposals out of economic self-interest. But the AMA remained coy. Its representative on the coalition, Dr. James H. Sammons, commented that the successful implementa-tion of the proposal was "a matter of degree and techniques." Obviously, AMA, a lobbying organization, is looking out for its member physicians. It is certain that doctors as a group will fight to preserve the status quo. A member of the federal panel, Dr. John Eisenberg of the University of Pennsylvania, reported, "The panel is examining how doctors are paid." But he added that "there is a limit to the amount of care that doctors can provide gratis. Doctors," he went on, "perceive that having a national health care system is not the same thing as government providing that care. The financing mechanism is under review more than the endemic causes and effects." His concern is for the methodology of practice related to finances. We must treat the causes simultaneously as we address the financing. Otherwise, we can find ourselves with another type of Medicare, thus adding additional money to an already costly system.

Major insurance companies are also facing tremendous losses. In 1988 Cigna, Prudential, Aetna, Metropolitan, and other insurers experienced deficits in the health care field despite their intention to embrace managed health care. These companies are trying to shift to the principles of managed health care, but they are keeping one leg, two arms, and their heads stuck in the indemnity rut. But if these large financial institutions can work effectively with business and government to reduce the total costs and establish as a priority efficiency and quality in health care, there is an even chance that this powerful triumvirate can bring about some form of legislative resolution to the health crisis.

Here are five ways in which business can make its health care outlays more productive. Business and government must develop rules of conduct from the medical community.

1. Have the hospital prove its real costs, not the ones created to maximize reimbursement.
2. Produce report cards on the outcome of the type of care purchased.
3. Don't pay for a hospital's past mistakes of overbuilding linked to high debt burden.
4. Ask for proof of increased efficiency, such as personnel costs and purchasing in ratio to patient care.
5. Accountability is a prerequisite to future costs. This accountability must be patient-care-related. Costs not related to patient care, such as other business ventures like pharmacies, durable medical equipment companies, or structural reorganization, should not be tolerated as hospital overhead.

CHAPTER ◆ ELEVEN

There's No Free Health Care for Consumers

Each year American employees are digging deeper into their pockets to cover their health needs. But for some reason, perhaps because they think the employer is paying for all of it, few workers, white- or blue-collar, seem aware of it. Typical pay stub deductions include income tax, Social Security, life and disability insurance, union dues if appropriate, "401K" contributions, and voluntary payments to the pension plan; with so many deductions, the one for health care is rarely noticed.

As coverage expands and inflation continues, "Employees are being asked to pay more of their own medical expenses," as Lance Tane, the consultant for the Wyatt Company, told *Business Insurance*. In its 1988 survey, Wyatt found that among the core group of 170 employers with comprehensive medical plans, 71 percent imposed a deductible of more than $100 in 1988, compared with 59 percent in 1986 and 45 percent in 1984. But the percentage of employees with deductibles of less than $100 fell to 1 percent in 1988, compared with 7 percent in 1986 and 21 percent in 1984.

Employers imposing a $100 deductible declined to 28 percent in 1988, against 34 percent in both 1986 and 1984. In other words, the employees' protection from burdensome health care costs substantially eroded in the five-year period.

Commenting on these rising deductibles, Tane stated that companies should consider even higher deductibles, perhaps as much as $1,000, or else link deductible levels to salary, as a handful of companies have already done.

Tane added, "When employees have a direct economic stake [through higher deductibles] in controlling health care costs, they tend to be better consumers of health care services." I don't agree, because patients do not order their own tests or procedures; but there's little doubt that health care and the assorted costs of a comprehensive health benefit package will become a major issue in management-labor negotiations.

Also, unions are beginning to recognize that employers are intensifying their efforts to reduce health costs by passing them on to their employees. The Communications Workers of America, recently defining six broad objectives in labor negotiations, devoted only one paragraph to wage increases but more than two pages to health care. Obviously, medical benefits for 500,000 workers are one of the most troublesome issues to iron out with management. Three years ago, the communications workers' demands for changes in health care coverage were strongly resisted by the NYNEX subsidiary of the American Telephone and Telegraph Company. The result was a two-week strike at NYNEX for health benefits. Recently SEPTA (Southeastern Pennsylvania Transportation Authority) narrowly averted a strike by a concession that indexed health care benefits to health care inflation.

In the teamsters' union, health care costs for 250,000 members amounts to 13 percent of wages, up from less than 10 percent six years ago. This growing bite from the workers' paycheck is certain to remain a pressing issue, and workers who have ignored the health care deduction will find that they have to pay more attention to it.

Two points must be made here. First, try as hard as they can, employers can only cut their commitments for employee health care so far. When their efforts to pass on an increasing portion of the costs meet opposition from their workers, it can lead to an impasse like the NYNEX strike. Or, more wisely, it can lead to a realization that the medical care delivery system needs a dramatic overhaul, and that the health insurance business needs to be taken over and operated by people who understand how this overhaul can be accomplished.

Second, Americans certainly need health care insurance, particularly when even a short hospital stay can cost many thousands of dollars and part of the cost must be absorbed by the recipients. How much is too much? Eight percent, 10 percent, 15 percent of one's gross pay? The point is debatable, at the least, and inconclusive as a general measure, at best.

But we must face the fact that if employers continue to receive large premium increases from the insurers, they will surely pass them on to their employees in the form of larger deductibles and increased copayments. The employee, in turn, will either have to absorb these deductibles or accept insufficient medical attention.

On the other hand, it would be unrealistic to look to the provider community—the hospitals, the physicians, and the professional laboratories—to reduce their fees. They will continue to be more creative in billing for services, especially as Medicare and Medicaid reduce their contributions to the health bill. And those costs will also be increased as inefficiency in the health care system takes its toll. New hospitals, for example, will default on their debt, especially those with tax-exempt status, because they were funded with the belief that government and industry would continue to reimburse hospitals in the same way indefinitely.

But no matter what the approach, the health care equation will be further exacerbated by the "graying" of America. Older citizens require more care and health costs will increase along with the percentage of Americans sixty years of age and older. Both past administrations and the current one have cut the rate of increase in the Medicare funding pool and have increasingly shifted costs to the Medicare recipient. The public's supplemental insurance premiums have continued to escalate, but the shift has not curtailed the country's total Medicare outlays.

So as the consumer finds himself digging deeper into his pockets to pay for his health needs and those of his family, he will need to protect himself.

The best any sensible, informed consumer can do is to shop for a comprehensive, affordable health plan with the lowest deductible and copayment. Don't be deluded by the "free $10,000 life insurance benefit." It's only a ploy to make you think you are getting something for very little. Insurance brokers can provide group life insurance much cheaper than health insurance so they ask you to buy a new package with less health care coverage and more life insurance. If you fall for that type of unfounded promise, you will be giving up more than you are getting. As a consumer, you should use a pencil, paper, and small calculator, and add up normal medical needs, such as a case of the flu, or healthy baby care, or annual checkups. These costs would easily run $800 a year. Think through your own experience and price out your exposure. There is a good feeling in having comprehensive protection.

This might be a good place to discuss U.S. Healthcare, because it provides quality health care on a very competitive basis.

We believe that U.S. Healthcare leads the way in consumer benefits by providing quality health care on a very competitive basis. It approaches provider negotiations with a clear sense of the reality of the situation, and with a complete understanding of the various billing mechanisms the provider community offers. It always tries to negotiate the most comprehensive, inclusive cost and to provide the American public with the best-quality care available. Accordingly, all the physicians who act as providers for the members must follow stringent guidelines and fully one-third of those who apply are rejected. Those accepted must be annually recertified.

Hospital administrators know that U.S. Healthcare will not

accept separate costs from synthetic corporations such as anesthesiology, radiology, pathology, cardiology, and so on and will only negotiate all-inclusive per diems. Consumers who purchase health care programs that besiege them with these innovative billing mechanisms find themselves subjected to numerous bills and various onerous copayments. Hospitals will send numerous separate bills from various departments. One bill would come from anesthesiology, another from radiology, another for medications, and so on. And it is not uncommon for some institutions to present a patient with as many as a dozen bills for hospital treatment. Some of these same hospitals use a dozen different computerized billing systems that are completely uncoordinated.

In addition, it appears that when various third-party administrators and insurance brokers encourage the employer to shift costs to the employee, they are openly exposing him to these manifold billing practices. The fact that the copayments and deductibles that result will prove a great burden to the individual doesn't seem to matter. That's why U.S. Healthcare spurns many of these separate and inflated payments.

The endless cost spiral that has afflicted employers and employees alike has spawned new responsibilities for health benefits managers in many corporations. One of their obligations has been to generate better understanding among workers as to their needs and options in medical insurance. This is discussed in a February 1989 article in *Board Briefing,* which is published for members of hospital and health care boards by Witt Associates. "Changes in health care environment have created a new role for the benefits manager in major companies—General Electric, Ford, Nestlé, NCR and many others," according to Allan Fine, senior associate. "Today's benefits managers are more skilled in negotiations, planning and data analysis than in the past, and chief executives increasingly hold them accountable for curtailing the rising spiral of health care costs," he said.

"Negotiating skills are needed to develop optimal arrangements with health care providers that hold down costs while offering choice to the employee. Planning skills are necessary to develop long-range strategies for health care cost containment. Data analysis skills are essential to handle the staggering amount of information provided by utilization review companies, insurance carriers and third-party administrators.

"Additionally," says Fine, "the benefits manager today combines the function of teacher, consultant and cheerleader for new ideas when communicating with employees on changes in the benefit plan. Cost containment efforts will be popular with employees if they perceive they are being given real choices, not limitations."

The last phrase is worth repeating, for it is necessary both to reduce costs and to keep the employees happy.

I visualize the following changes:

◆ Employers will move toward fixed-contribution schedules rather than fixed-benefit plans. Employers will allow employees to decide whether they want to spend more for a greater selection or exchange flexibility for more coverage.

◆ Many indemnity insurance companies will attempt to lead employers to fully insured benefit programs and away from the uninsured programs typical of the last decade. As a result, employers will realize that they can no longer afford the perceived modest savings that come with the risk of spiraling costs for unmanaged health care and administration.

◆ Consumers will purchase more effective cost-containment programs that reduce costs rather than create them.

◆ The federal government will consider some sort of legislative guarantee of minimum tax-deductible benefit levels to protect employees from "shifting the shaft," or shifting the burden of absorbing the cost increases from employers to employees.

In addition, as costs rise and there are new technological breakthroughs, we will have to make some practical decisions.

They will involve such things as the turmoil in Blue Cross plans. In 1988 there were seventy-seven Blue Cross plans in operation, which produced a loss of $900 million as of June. The national Blue Cross predicted that the loss could reach $1.2 billion in 1989. Only eleven of the seventy-seven plans reported gains and sixty-six had losses for the first six months. It was certainly a barometer of what the fee-for-service system can do to an insuring entity.

Society will have to decide how best to handle lawyers and the legal system in terms of the wealth of litigation. There is no question that our system is being much abused—"ripped off" may be a more apt term—by lawyers practicing personal injury law. The cost added by the litigious monster that we have spawned adds great costs not only to medical fees but to almost every product and service in our economy.

What of those consumers who purchase their own health care insurance? From a cost or inflationary standpoint, they are not doing as well as the company employee. The cost of purchasing one's own health care is growing at about 20 percent a year for those individuals—about double the company employee's cost. These stand alone, unrepresented.

One cannot ignore perception and its effect. As Robert J. Blendon of the Harvard University School of Public Health wrote in the January 1989 issue of the *Journal of the American Medical Association,* analyzing seventy-five national opinion polls conducted between 1966 and 1987: "Poll trends highlight a growing dilemma for the nation's health care leaders. On one hand, costs, competition and bed occupancy are pressuring medical care to become more businesslike and commercial. On the other hand, if medicine follows this route, it risks losing the public's trust in the profession's views of what constitutes quality of care, and, sometime in the future, there may be a strong regulatory backlash."

There's no free lunch for consumers—or anyone else.

CHAPTER TWELVE

Preventive Health Care, or the Best of Remedies

Among society's many role models, one of the most salutary would be the health enthusiast or advocate, whether it's Kurt Thomas, the Olympic gymnast; Jane Fonda, the actress with her exercise and diet regimen; or Oprah Winfrey, the TV talk show hostess who shed seemingly countless pounds. Not that any of these are the most sterling examples; but a role model offers us positive opportunities, even if it is just the neighbor who is out every morning, rain or shine, jogging as we leave for work.

There's no doubt that the quality of our life today is greatly dependent upon hereditary factors and environmental and mental attitudes. Yet there seems to be endless and futile debate about why some of us are healthier than others and why some Americans are constantly in and out of doctors' offices and hospitals, and why we constantly dose ourselves with all manner of medications.

A preventive health care program can be developed by finding and emulating a health-advocate role model and adhering to habits that will maintain a healthy body. Obviously, we cannot influence heredity, but we can influence environmental factors and we can, to a great degree, influence our state of mind.

One doesn't have to look very far to find America's unhealthy habits. We ingest tons of animal fats and sugar products, washed down by drinks full of a variety of chemicals sweetened and colored to give instant gratification. We still ingest tremendous amounts of tobacco and further aggravate our bodies with alcohol. Efforts to neutralize these effects present us with a ludicrous situation. American television is filled with beer and fast-food commercials mingled with commercials plugging the instant use of antacids and Alka-Seltzer–type products to soothe our irritated stomachs.

With the human body subjected to the type of punishment that we put it through, it is little wonder that our health care bills are as high as they are. To correct our self-imposed ills and discomforts, we swallow pills, tonics, and potions, hopefully dispensed by physicians eager to cure us and return us to a state of health. Where is our sense of self-discipline, our role models, our natural inclination for self-protection?

We are certainly subjected to pressures in our work life and family life; minimizing abuse to our bodies could help us maintain our health.

It is hardly the purpose of this chapter to offer a long, detailed explanation of why Americans suffer from so many ills. Its purpose instead is to prompt all of us to think about how our dietary and other habits really hurt us and how they influence the cost of health care. In my view, this book would not be complete in tackling the big subject of healing our health care system if we did not talk about how we can take command of healing ourselves.

Prevention is obviously a prime factor in reducing our health care bills, but it is certainly not a uniform goal, judging from the kinds of drugs most Americans take. Most of them are remedies for illnesses we already suffer. Periodically, the American drug industry lists the top ten drugs and among them are tranquilizers, ulcer medication, headache pills, pain tablets, heart and blood-pressure medications, and diabetic medication.

American medicine has come a long way and continues to make progress in building greater understanding of how the human body works and how to treat its malfunctions. We now understand genes and how they influence our behavior and our health. However, in the most recent decades, we have become a society that is overtreated, overmedicated, overtested, and is less responsible for its own health than ever before.

Let's examine a typical case of low-back pain and the manner in which it is treated in a modern metropolitan city.

An individual experiences low-back pain, a painful muscle spasm that prevents him from performing normal, daily functions. Most low-back pain is induced by stress, lack of exercise, or chronic tension. Our subject with the sore back may go to an emergency room because of the pain and disability or may be too frightened to move. This is the usual scenario: The physician takes a history and examination of the patient, orders an X-ray, possibly a CAT scan, and writes prescriptions for a muscle relaxant and possibly pain medication. This experience could cost the patient or the patient's insurance company several hundred dollars. But probably all the patient needs is some bed rest, hot showers, aspirin tablets, and some personal introspection on what is causing his or her back to act up.

If it is a question of stress at the workplace or in the home, there are methods that people can adopt to ease the tension, such as taking regular breaks or taking a walk. A break usually means a brief change of environment, and a brisk walk may help to relax and even develop back muscles. Our subject may further complain of that chronic back problem because of his or her lifestyle, and being placed in a back brace may only exacerbate the problem.

In fact, there are some situations in which the patient may even be hospitalized and placed in traction. But if you press them hard enough, most orthopedists will admit that normal traction utilized in the hospital is worthless except for making an admitting diagnosis and placing the patient in a hospital bed. This type of treatment is costly, ineffective, and usually leads to a recurrence.

We can cure this condition in many other ways—exercise, relaxation, and therapy work wonders when no pathology exists.

Let's now take an individual who is really ill and may have diabetes. The diabetic can be helped greatly by appropriate dietary habits and adequate exercise, and by the appropriate use of hypoglycemics or insulin, depending upon how the particular physician treats the patient.

However, many cases of diabetic complications are worsened because the individual has not been properly educated about good health habits and proper life-style. That is a basic need that every doctor must address in treating a diabetic.

In general, we all must learn which foods can help us heal ourselves and make our bodies fit. These include whole-grain cereals, fresh fruit and vegetables, and unadulterated foods. We should spurn simple sugars, candy, ice cream, and fast-food snacks. Many times, some or all of these are used primarily for gratification to relieve boredom or stress but only result in weight gain and excessive salt and sugar intake. In short, they are not anything we would ingest if we considered the havoc they can create within our bodies.

Quite a few years ago, Nathan Pritikin introduced Americans to a fat-free diet combined with an exercise program. Initially, many internists and cardiologists pooh-poohed this regimen. But today it has become the type of standard diet that many Americans sooner or later embrace to prevent arteriosclerosis, to lower their blood pressure, to achieve weight loss. Our workplace and school cafeterias all make available to us a selection of salads, fruits, vegetables, and other foods that can help to reduce health care disorders.

Furthermore, it goes without saying that overmedication and overtreatment are not the road to a healthy, enjoyable existence. Appropriate checkups and early diagnosis of life-threatening illnesses can yield a higher cure rate and help to save lives. But we have become a society accustomed to quick, defensive, instant, and expensive treatment.

Perhaps the subject compels us to be candid, even brutally so.

Our Medicare patient population is a sad example of how patients, physicians, and hospitals all participate in the further abuse of an already overutilized and overbilled health care system. Many elderly people who are bored have found that a visit to the doctor, or having medical treatment elsewhere, is a way to fill up time. Thus, the visit to the cardiologist, podiatrist, internist, or other type of physician becomes part of a calendar-filling series of activities that are financed in great part by our federal government.

This type of misbehavior is not only pathetic, it is also shocking when one visits a neighborhood pharmacy and watches some of the elderly approach the pharmacist with a plastic bag filled with a variety of medications, often costing them hundreds of dollars a month at the expense of their food needs and social life. Often, many of these drugs are contraindicated and are being prescribed by three or four different physicians without the coordination of a family physician.

In essence, preventive health care must start with individuals taking charge of their own bodies and health. And prevention begins with simple, basic, commonsense health habits:

◆ Get an ample amount of sleep.

◆ Set aside enough time for a run or some other exercise that can reduce stress.

◆ Reduce or fully eliminate your dependence upon caffeine and sweetened, carbonated drinks.

◆ Reduce the amount of animal fat you eat. Substitute cereals, vegetables, and fresh fruit.

◆ Do not use tobacco in any form.

◆ Reduce the amount of alcohol you drink. A little wine is OK, but excessive alcohol is not good.

◆ Develop a positive mental attitude.

♦ Rid yourself and your body of dependency on drugs.

♦ Develop a good, informed relationship with your family doctor.

♦ Take charge of your medical treatment, at least to the extent that you are not confused by it and are reassured that it is proper and on track. Insist that your questions be clarified.

♦ Research the medical delivery system that you are going to use, such as the physicians, the laboratory, the hospital, the hospital staff, and comparative costs and related health issues. (The selection of a good medical plan is discussed in detail in Chapter 13.)

♦ Women should have an annual Pap test and women over thirty-five should have mammograms, coordinated with self-administered breast examinations.

♦ Men should have yearly examinations that include electrocardiograms, and rectal and occult blood studies to detect early colon and rectum cancer.

♦ Check weight, blood pressure, and cholesterol count. Most important, read articles on health care and maintenance. Become a student of good dietary habits. Read magazines and newspapers that give helpful health hints. Your own health care plan and family physician are reliable sources, along with the Government Printing Office, which has health care literature.

But, as always, one is on one's own. If you adopt good health habits, you will gain self-respect. You might even become your own role model—or one for your family or friends.

CHAPTER THIRTEEN

Common Sense
for a Common Cause

If all else fails, try common sense.

You've heard that before, of course, but I heartily endorse it. Any business principle that brings cost-effective and quality results almost always has simple common sense at its core. Let me enunciate a few basic principles involved in any effort to improve our health care system.

Principle 1

We can assess quantity and quality of hospital performance by comparing their costs and their procedure rates.

In 1989, using very conservative estimates, the cost of health insurance will increase at least 21 to 22 percent across the board. This trend will continue into the 1990s. Whether self-funded or insured, the average employer should know where these increases come from. Estimates show that 6.3 percent of the increase emanated from cost shifting; 3.5 percent came from increased utilization; 7.1 percent from medical inflation; 0.3 percent for malpractice insurance; 2.4 percent for technology; and 1.9 percent from catastrophic causes. America will enter the 1990s with health care costs reaching 12 percent of the GNP. As of this printing there are health care experts predicting health care costs reaching 15 percent of the GNP by the year 2000. The buying public, too, should recognize that there are great differences in the same procedures among competing hospitals in the area. Here are a few examples:

	Hospital A	Hospital B	Hospital C	Hospital D
CHEST PAIN	$1,774	$2,862	$3,911	$3,694
CHOLECYSTECTOMY	2,687	6,363	8,109	8,452
VAGINAL DELIVERY	2,075	3,304	4,589	3,802
C-SECTION	2,475	4,633	6,385	5,288

Armed with this type of competitive information, we can assess quality and quantity because the number of cases performed in a hospital by physicians does directly affect the quality. The more procedures a hospital has, the better are its outcome statistics.

Principle 2

This evaluation also leads us to conclude that our country needs a national medical-quality-assurance program. We don't have one, strange as it may seem.

The recent suggestions for universal health insurance are based upon providing a minimum level of health insurance at a minimum cost. But it has been estimated that between 25 to 40 percent of the medical care delivery in this system is inappropriate. Inappropriate care increases the cost of health care without producing any health care benefits.

But a good quality-assurance program could improve the incidence of appropriate utilization. It could thereby improve the quality of care being provided to the nation's consumers and at the same time help cut health care costs. In our current system, when a physician becomes licensed and fulfills his license requirements, his license is renewed annually after paying a nominal fee. He participates in the Medicare and Medicaid programs by indicating that he wishes to participate. Generally, he remains in the programs unless it can be proved that he has demonstrated fraud or flagrant abuse. There is no attempt to assess his quality of care before renewing his license or allowing him to continue his participation in Medicare or Medicaid. If you become sick, you go to a doctor, a diagnosis is made, and treatment is rendered; the doctor's quality of delivery is generally not considered.

Here's a simple checklist that we can use ourselves—or the country could adopt—to determine medical appropriateness:

♦ Was the time it took to get an appointment with the doctor suitable for the complaint?

♦ Was the length of time needed to make a diagnosis appropriate?

♦ Were the proper tests ordered?

♦ Were the tests accurately reported?

♦ Was the treatment correct?

♦ Were there complications resulting from the treatment?

♦ Was the outcome reasonable?

♦ Was the treating facility appropriate for the condition?

♦ Was the cost for the treatment competitive with that given to other similarly treated patients across the country?

If there is currently a method of measuring the quality of care, why should it not be available to everyone? U.S. Healthcare has such a method and the public at large should receive a similar benefit.

An actual quality-assurance program patterned after U.S. Healthcare's would yield these benefits: It would be broadly applied to the private sector; it would not require reorganizing the present delivery system. There are good quality-assurance programs in the managed-care sector, but these are associated with staff models and would not be applicable on a broad basis, such as physicians practicing in individual independent offices. Staff model physicians are employees, and as such their charts and methods of practice can be standardized.

Principle 3

U.S. Healthcare's program has been applied entirely in a private-practice setting; and it could be used as a functional model for managed health care. The program utilizes 2,300 primary physicians, 10,000 specialists, and currently covers over 1 million members. The system strikes a balance between quality and appropriateness of care and offers choice as to the delivery system, bringing quality assurance into the doctor's office, not just the hospital. It assesses the quality of the entire medical experience from home to office to hospital to pharmacy. It includes a large data base covering laboratory, radiology, and other ancillary services. Licensure, staff privileges to practice in certain hospitals, and participation in federal and state programs such as Medicare and Medicaid are integrated into ongoing data bases.

The system attacks the question of the quality of medical care by making all providers of health care measurable and accountable to the review program. There has been much said, and much more will be said, about incentive programs, particularly relating to physicians. Most of the focus has been on criticism of incentive programs and very little attention has been directed toward the positive results of incentives, which when linked to positive quality-control standards and good supervision by peers, will result in better-quality care. I believe that when individuals are paid to do more, they will do more. If they are paid to do less, they will refer more to other physicians and therefore increase the costs, as well as the amount of unnecessary care.

Principle 4

The best way of improving our health care system is to establish a scorecard on each health care provider, and I propose the development of categories or tiers of care.

The categories of practitioners would be broad, depending upon similarities of practice, and points of comparison would include such issues as incidence of infection after surgical procedures or length of stay for hospitalized patients compared with regional or national statistics. The categories would be made up of quality-assurance measurements combined with appropriateness of care and utilization assessments.

In U.S. Healthcare's quality-assurance program, this categorization is linked directly to compensation of the primary care physician. In regard to specialist physicians, it is tied to their recertification and prevents them from continuing in the plan if they do not meet recertification criteria. In an operating quality-assurance program, categorization is used in many different ways:

◆ It is tied to participation in both the Medicare and Medicaid programs.

◆ It could be tied to license renewal with or without restrictions. States have the right to limit the medical practice of physicians.

◆ It could be tied to the appropriateness of restricted or unrestricted hospital stays.

◆ It could include publication of category listing similar to the Health Care Financing Agency's publishing of hospital death rates.

◆ It could award certificates for display along with the medical license and other credentials.

◆ It could be tied to maintenance of satisfactory society membership—physicians who belong to medical societies are more conscious of their peers than those that don't.

◆ It could be tied to modification of the level of malpractice premiums.

And the quality-assurance measurement could include:

◆ Adherence to established standards of care.

◆ Scoring of patients' questionnaires. This would assess the subjective impression of the doctor's patient as to the quality of the service.

◆ Quality of recordkeeping.

◆ Outcome of analysis for frequent procedures such as:
—Incidence of infections after surgical procedures.
—Incidence of readmission within a set time after discharge.
—Incidence of bleeding requiring transfusions after surgical procedure.
—Length of stay in hospitals compared to the norm.

◆ Patient grievances, categorized, measured, and used for reference.

The appropriateness-of-care assessments would also include a percentage of procedures performed in the appropriate manner when compared to standards of appropriateness set by recognized and accepted experts. Also measured would be the percentage of appropriate hospital admissions compared to established standard recommendations for treatment when compared to mandatory second-opinion situations, and the appropriate use of consultants.

These are some commonsense approaches that can be developed by the public, physicians, and regulatory agencies, and they can be linked to each other. It is my firm belief that this will not only improve the quality but decrease the cost of care. And, importantly, these report cards for care, which will become part of the basis for choosing and paying a physician, a health plan, an insurance company, a hospital, or ancillary services, will readily be made available to the public.

Principle 5

Since we are stressing common sense, in addition to our own preventive steps we should take certain precautions:

♦ Don't rely solely on an insurance broker. He may choose a plan or a product that is best for his bottom line, not yours.

♦ Don't rely solely on your employee benefits officer. The company's chief executive officer, chief financial officer, and representatives from the employee ranks should also be involved. Health care benefits are too costly not to be analyzed by the best minds in the company.

♦ Don't allow the ease of administration to determine your company's benefits. Too often, employee benefits representatives will choose a quickly accessible product rather than one that may require more work and scrutiny. Don't allow your personal physician to influence your choice—his or her fee-for-service mentality may prejudice the recommendation. Your physician should be a source of information, not the advisor for your choice of health plan.

Principle 6

Constant awareness is essential. To achieve it, try these recommendations:

♦ Shop your benefit plan annually.

♦ If you are an employer or executive, walk in your employee's shoes. See how much protection, service, and costs will accrue to them.

◆ Be sure you have a choice among plans or some direct method of negotiating and selecting medical providers. Do not allow yourself to be completely removed from the selection of physician or hospital, because the choice could be more costly and the outcome poorer than you desire.

◆ Do not accept risk. If you are an executive with lots of other responsibilities on your back, let experienced professionals advise you. Administrative service only, employee preference option, and other self-insurance programs will ultimately cost you more, not less. Your loss ratio plus your administrative fees can well surpass most fixed premiums.

◆ Set up budgets and work hard to stay within them. Don't be afraid to shop selectively and send out RFPs (requests for proposals) to find the designs or program with which you are most comfortable.

◆ Educate yourself in the comparative performances of insurance companies, HMOs, PPOs, EPOs, third-party administrators, utilization review companies, hospital costs, physician's costs and report cards, and physician's costs and performances for which you should develop report cards.

◆ Hold your insurer accountable. Maintain a competitive stance. Do not turn over all of your insurance coverage to one broker or to one company. Ask your insurer for the following statistical information: member surveys; member grievances; physician and hospital certification and recertification; quality assurance performance; loss ratios; general administrative costs; preventive programs; and coordination of benefit performance.

Aside from this, let me share with you U.S. Healthcare's 1988 statistics, which we make available to our employers as an indication of how quantity and quality of health care can be ranked.

In 1988 U.S. Healthcare's members had 2,774,134 primary

care visits. They had 143,000 Pap smears, and of those 90 percent were Class I, 7.4 percent were Class II, 1.2 percent were Class III, and 0.04 percent were Class IV. (Briefly, these classes can be defined as: Class I, normal; Class II, negative for malignant cells with some atypical cells that may indicate infection or inflammation; Class III, more atypical cells but not necessarily malignant cells; Class IV, malignant cells present.) We conducted surveys of members concerning quality of care in primary care offices, with the total number of surveys being 604,000. We recertified 1,212 offices. We reviewed 4,400 hospitals' record reviews. The company reviewed 36,223 ambulatory records. U.S. Healthcare performed 1,611,000 blood tests using modern clinical laboratory procedure in a quality laboratory.

In addition, the company received written grievances for primary care at the rate of 0.03 percent. The professional service coordinator for our HMOs in Pennsylvania and New Jersey made 6,495 visits. Medical director site visits in both states alone totaled 593. About 600,000 members were surveyed and 86.7 percent said they would recommend their primary care physician to a friend. During the year, the company filled 2,623,000 prescriptions. The number of visits of children in their first twenty-four months to primary care doctors, including well-baby visits, totaled 223,696.

Obviously, this type of statistical base is quite valuable in measuring both the quality and quantity of health care. It is the result of a commonsense, quantitative approach which has led to success for our company and can surely lead to positive results for the country at large. We offer our experience to be used, tested, fully examined, and replicated. I and my company stand behind this offer of help to any organization or company that wishes to take advantage of it.

At the outset of this chapter, I suggested that if all else fails, try common sense. But what if common sense fails? Then we are in much worse shape in this country than we should be.

CHAPTER FOURTEEN

Typical Questions, Some Untypical Answers

One of America's greatest strengths is its ability to change and its endless flexibility. So it should be with our troubled health care system. But to change it, some hard questions must be asked and answered, such as:

How much health care can the United States afford?

As it ponders its priorities, our society will answer this from the standpoint of its real value system. How much is an effective American health care system worth? The percentage of our gross national product that we allocate for it will depend upon such questions as "What do we get for our investment in the health care system?" and "How should other resources such as those for education, housing, defense, and so on be allocated?" And the puzzle of why we waste 20 percent of our health care costs should certainly be factored into it. The competition created for different and opposing resources will help us decide how much health care we can afford.

Should the health care system be reorganized?

Yes. We need a coordinated system in which the fragmented components are joined for overall benefit. The new program must be an insurer, producer, and provider of health care. In other words, the companies or organizations providing the insurance should integrate all the important components of health care. Competing factions add to costs and often do not provide coordinated care.

Do we want the federal government to intervene?

Unfortunately, the federal government must intervene but in a manner that ensures that public policy becomes one of improving quality, improving access, and reducing overall costs.

Why do physicians favor the Canadian system of health care as an alternative?

Federal dollars in Canada are apportioned to the provinces, where local budgets are set up. Fees are negotiated on a local level. Physicians can negotiate as a group for their fees. Physicians feel more comfortable when they have negotiating ability with the third-party payer.

Should research and education be funded separately from patient care?

Yes. As a nation, we must make sure that education in all forms is funded separately. Why? Because it is counterproductive to force society to pay hidden taxes in the form of more expensive health care. Soon after starting practice, physicians should begin to repay the cost of their medical education and end their obligations within fifteen years.

What type of organization can best insure Americans' health care?

An organization in which decision-making is shared by health care leaders with the overall authority to carry out public policy that measures quality, quantity, and accessibility.

How should we break up the oligarchies?

Hospitals' and Blue Cross's dominance are counterproductive to both effective quality and cost-efficiency. The influence that hospitals and Blue Cross have in many areas of the United States, such as in Pittsburgh, have created very expensive care. The Justice Department must study these oligarchies for antitrust violations, break them up, and permit competition.

Should the legal system be altered to allow health care reform?

Yes. The nation's legal system contributes very heavily to high costs. It compels physicians to practice a sort of defensive form of medicine because lawyers are constantly stalking medical practices looking for opportunities to sue doctors. If physicians are guaranteed a strong peer review of quality and behavior, they, and we, will have a defense against such lawyers. If successful, we can beat them off and send them packing to seek other areas in our society for malpractice litigation. Another area of cost reform in the legal system involves personal injury cases. These arise from loopholes in our health care system. These must be closed to curb lawyers from referring patients to doctors who practice medicine in ways that increase medical bills and lead to waste because of unneeded care.

How important are quality and accountability?

It no longer suffices to say that we have quality care. We must provide accountability through quantitative standards of measuring performance. In the next decade, quality will emerge as a paramount area of importance in providing reduced cost and improved quality. In the last chapter of this book, I will dwell in great detail on how both quality and accountability will bring about a reduction of costs and expand health care benefits to many more

Americans. The need to achieve accountability in quantitative terms is vital.

Why is Great Britain modifying its health care system? Can we learn from that country?

Great Britain is in dire need of modernizing and improving the infrastructure of its health care delivery system. (See Chapter 7.) Under the universal health system, relatively little money has been expended on building new hospitals and on improving the physical plants in general. Because of the system's inadequacies in terms of finance and service, Great Britain is reaching into the private sector to attempt to modify its national health care system. What we can learn from it, in my opinion, is that socialized medicine in itself creates as many problems as it solves. Yet, at the same time, a recent poll by Louis Harris and Associates found that Americans are more dissatisfied with their health care system than either Canadians or Britons, despite the higher outlays for health care in this country. According to the survey, 89 percent of Americans said that their health care system needed fundamental changes; 61 percent said that they would exchange the American system for the Canadian model; and 29 percent favored the American system. Sixty-nine percent of Britons said that they wanted extensive changes in their system, but only 12 percent said that they preferred the American model.

Can our hospitals be helped?

Americans were less likely than Britons or Canadians to say that they were satisfied with the hospital stays or physicians' office visits during their previous year, according to the poll. The growing dissatisfaction with our system always singles out hospitals. But hospitals can be helped in the following ways:

♦ Unnecessary layers of administrative staff can be eliminated. Use of consultants also can be eliminated or greatly reduced. Only those costs that are directly patient-care-related should be budgeted. All extraneous, associated activities that add costs to the hospital budget, such as those layers of corporate subsidiaries aimed at venturing into far-flung business ventures, can be cast aside. Hospitals and hospital administrators who envision themselves as entrepreneurs miss one big fact—that is, entrepreneurs take *risks.*

◆ Strong individuals should be hired to manage hospitals but at the same time they should be relegated to the role of "benevolent dictator." They should be given authority, but it should be controlled. Those individuals should develop a five-year growth plan to improve the hospital's patient care and support.

◆ Each hospital must establish its own mission and raison d'être. Some should be closed and others saved in order to better serve society. Purchasing must come under a microscope. I contend that the cost of purchasing can be cut at least 10 percent by creating effective controls, by reducing waste, and by cutting general administrative costs. Hospitals should be used seven days a week. It is absolutely silly and wasteful to fund a hospital, staff it properly, but not use it on Saturdays and Sundays. Methods must also be developed to use the hospital's operating rooms, X-ray facilities, and laboratories on weekends.

How do we enlist the help of the physician community?

Physicians will cooperate and support positive change if they see it leading to an improvement in the economics and quality of American health care. If they perceive that the common good is served while their own individuality is preserved and they can benefit from an improved, strengthened medical system, they will become equal partners in the more beneficial environment. The simple fact is that doctors must be included and involved in the overall strategy of a changed system. They must be shown how their professional and personal conduct really influence patient care and costs in their own practice and in hospitals.

Will this voluntary effort work?

Indeed it will, even though no voluntary effort by either physicians or hospitals to date has proved effective. I am convinced that all our efforts to improve our health care system need voluntary cooperation. But those efforts will only succeed when doctors realize they are being scrutinized and held accountable for how effective their performance is and clearly understand what their performance thresholds should be.

What's driving the insurance industry toward managed health care?

The insurance industry has been pummeled by high medical costs through their indemnity insurance entities. Those are clearly out of control. The insurance industry recognizes that with the reduction of Medicare reimbursement and the competition between indemnity insurance companies and managed health care systems, the hospital industry and the physician communities are billing full fee-for-service to the indemnity insurance carriers. Thus, they have no choice if they want to stay in the health care business but to develop alternative programs that are managed health care. However, to date many insurance companies are totally exiting the health care industry. The only way they can remain is through a managed health care product.

What happened to the catastrophic illness legislation called the Medicare Catastrophic Coverage Act of 1988 (H.R. 2470)?

The catastrophic illness legislation, repealed only sixteen months after its passage, ostensibly would have expanded Medicare coverage of high medical costs. It really was a means to test benefits because it was linked to payments of income. For approximately 40 percent of the Medicare enrollees, the plan had a mandatory maximum annual premium of $800, and this created a tremendous protest from the Medicare community. The House was unwavering in its call for repeal, and the vote was carried by a wide margin. The Senate, however, tried to salvage portions of the program. The Senate compromise basically would have eliminated the surtax and preserved the modest benefit package, though it eliminated the most costly nursing home and prescription drug coverage. The Bush administration only offered this bill lukewarm support. The executive branch was more interested in preserving the $5 billion of premium already collected than in maintaining the benefits. Only a few expanded programs in the bill's Medicaid sections remained after the final vote to repeal. Gone were the Medicare provisions. Under the compromise, for physician visits there would have been a return to the previous coverage, which was to limit payment to 80% of customary and reasonable charges after the beneficiary pays $75 of annual deductibles. The coverage for prescription drugs would not have any increased benefits. Nursing home care would return to a plan for the payment of one hundred days of post-hospital care, as was the case in 1988, when the patients paid coinsurance charges of $67.50 per day for twenty-one to one hundred days. The patient had to spend at least three days in the hospital prior to admission. The mammography benefit would have been retained as it was in the Catastrophic Coverage Act, but not in the previous Medicare Act. There would be no addition to home care coverage, and hospital care would return to previous coverage, which was up to ninety days for illness with a $540 deductible which would be increased annually. Patients were required to make copayments of $135 a day in 1988 for days sixty-one through ninety, with a lifetime reserve of sixty days of coverage with daily copayment charges of $278. Those benefits, however necessary to protect the Medicare community, disappeared in the furor and with the passage of the repeal legislation, H.R.3607.

Why is Medicare a major social problem today?

It would have been impossible for President Lyndon B. Johnson, in whose administration Medicare was enacted, to ever have forecast its total cost. Fundamentally, the economics are wrong. But the reason it has become a social problem is because the government is trying to control costs by shifting back much of that responsibility to the Medicare recipient. Therefore, many people on fixed incomes find themselves absorbing much more of the costs than they had previously anticipated. In addition, many hospitals had built major additions or new hospitals, assuming large debt on the assumption that Medicare reimbursement would go on forever. This has put them in a precarious position and much of their operating costs are being eaten up in paying both the debt and the interest on tax-free financing.

How can the average American make sure he or she is getting appropriate care?

The health care community must issue report cards. These can be one element whereby an individual can review the relative merits of a provider against those of others in a community. Second, a patient should have the right of full access to the health care plan. The plan must be staffed with knowledgeable individuals who can help provide guidance and answer questions on one's health care. And the average American must have a medical ombudsman who can help oversee and scrutinize the quality and quantity of care that he or she is getting.

How can the various alternative health plans be evaluated?

The Delivery of Care

◆ What is the model type—individual practice association or group model, where doctors practice in groups?

◆ Is care readily accessible?

◆ Emergency coverage. Is it covered? And in what manner?

Quality-of-Care Assessment

◆ Does the plan have the ability to positively influence medical providers' practice patterns? If so, how?

◆ Member surveys: Are they consistently conducted and how are they used?

Cost Management

◆ Does the plan have the ability to negotiate advantageous provider contracts?

◆ Utilization monitoring and control: Is it performed?

◆ Innovative provider reimbursement systems: Does the plan have experience and success in negotiating favorable contracts?

◆ Alternative care programs.

Financial Stability

◆ Strong balance sheet for several years for managed health care plans.

◆ Historical positive membership growth pattern.

Leadership

◆ Innovative programs in prevention and wellness.

◆ Medical recognition: Does the plan have a positive reputation?

Employee Satisfaction

◆ Comprehensive medical care assured throughout the community.

◆ Can you get access to nationally recognized institutions?

◆ Health screening and early detection such as cancer screening, occult blood studies, mammograms, and cholesterol screening.

◆ Reasonable cost.

Employer Satisfaction

◆ Premium-rate stability.

◆ Utilization reporting.

◆ Anticipation of and responsiveness to employer needs.

What should the federal government do about Medicare?

Medicare should be reshaped into what it was meant to be—a hybrid between government and private enterprise. We need the government to intervene with the regulatory clout similar to federal qualifications for HMOs and also to provide regulatory control over the provider community. Insurance companies must meet strict quality standards of medical delivery. Furthermore, we must provide incentives for providers and Medicare members to obtain efficiency and effectiveness. Health care costs will continue to rise until the federal government becomes involved in regulating benefits, quality, and costs.

What's the future for the American health care system?

It will become a partnership among government, business, medical providers, and the American people. The government will mandate certain basic benefits for insurance carriers, managed-care companies, and for employers. A tax credit will be issued for health care that meets certain standards. Quality will be used as a method of measurement. Physicians' fees will be standardized and hospitals will become more efficient, better-operated facilities. Improved hospital management will intensify competition. This, in turn, will improve services and patient satisfaction. If all this happens—and I think it will—the system will be strengthened and its costs will stabilize.

CHAPTER FIFTEEN

A Scenario
That Will Work

"He flung himself from the room, flung himself upon his horse and rode madly off in all directions," Stephen Leacock once wrote. Sometimes I think that this quote from the witty but almost forgotten Canadian humorist aptly describes the diverse, uncoordinated remedies that our national health leaders dream up to heal our system's ills.

Sadly, the missing quotient in many of these programs is a sense of practicality and workability. For example, for our insurance and provider communities to boast about quality is simply not enough. We must be able to measure and then approve accountability. Quality must be graded in quantitative terms, or it means very little in our workaday world.

As I review all that I have discussed in these pages so far, it seems that it has all been a setting of the stage, if you will, for what I will propose in these final pages. It is a scenario that presents all the players on the health care scene with a pragmatic means of solving many of their problems.

What I propose are standards of quantitative measurement to

compare levels of quality in health care delivery. In our world of desktop computers, personal computers, lap-top computers, and voice-activated computers, as well as the new horizons of optical scanning, the technology certainly exists for us to develop standardized medical protocols on quantity and quality that can be used in both the ambulatory and hospital sectors. They will reveal in clear, uncontestable terms the actual performance of our system. They will present the results of efforts by a broad-based group of quality physicians and medical administrators. They will include the findings of actuaries, statisticians, financial planners, and others. All this data will help us develop acceptable norms and standards of health care in our country.

I am proposing a concept in which we should be able to accept only quality care that meets acceptable measures of performance.

By establishing this accurate form of medical accountability and reporting, we should be able to accomplish several goals. One is the improvement of quality. Another is to provide a form of control over the 20 percent or more of unnecessary health care. A third will be a strong means of defending the medical community against the proliferating, litigious segment of our society, which we have fostered largely by ignoring it. And finally, we can achieve an overall reduction of costs.

With this measure, physicians thus held to a higher level of accountability will be convinced not to practice superfluous, unnecessary procedures and treatments because their performance will be reviewed and scrutinized by their peers. Inevitably, the medical community must take an active, aggressive role in peer review. Individuals who don't meet the standards simply will not be allowed to practice, nor will institutions that do not perform. Thus, the medical community will be able to police itself and reduce the number of malpractice claims and injury cases. Lawyers will find it much harder to influence the practice and methods in which physicians treat patients referred by lawyers. Lawyers, in order to meet insurance payment thresholds, refer clients to physicians who specialize in personal injury cases.

This new, increased peer review will be linked to standardized recordkeeping, as well as a high degree of electronic data transfer, and will result in improved care of health in all levels of American society. It will also improve necessary care and will increase the availability of physicians and hospitals who are presently squandering their resources and time in providing unnecessary care. Just think for a moment about how this accountability and peer review will relieve physicians' concerns about practicing defensive medicine and also reduce that type of practice. Furthermore, malpractice premiums will be reduced as the litigious trend subsides.

I see the government, as these reforms take hold, passing legislation that will provide for companies and individuals to purchase only health care programs that meet the accountability levels. Companies, in turn, will only be allowed to take tax deductions when their programs provide this accountability standard. The federal government will benefit from a dramatic lowering of the cost of Medicare and Medicaid and the reduction of the federal deficit, while ensuring a healthier nation. Obviously, the United States is stronger and more viable when its resources aren't squandered. Conversely, we are weakened when we tolerate the misuse of any valuable assets.

By reviewing the outcome data of a variety of reports that are made available to them, businesses will benefit. They will purchase only health care that meets the measurement standard, which is acceptable to the government and to the medical profession. As a result, they will be able to use their resources to purchase a more competitive level of care.

If it functions properly, the new system will have a double-barreled benefit. Report cards on physicians, hospitals, insurance companies, and HMOs will enable companies to cut their costs and to pare at least 20 percent of their care, which has been unnecessary. These reductions in savings can be directed to provide health care for the 37 million Americans who have no appropriate insurance today and for the 16 million who have substandard care because of soaring health costs.

The provider community will surely become an active force in policing itself. The insurance community will join with its actuaries, financial staffs, and physicians to measure the appropriateness of levels of care. New technology will be adopted to improve quality. The newer technology will reduce the number of invasive procedures and can help to reduce costs.

Unquestionably, we can obtain noninvasive procedures when we have the ability to reduce costs. Then the appropriateness of the use of, say, lithotripsy and the cost of other medical procedures will be compared to the actual equipment cost plus the resources needed to prepare the patient for the procedure. Unfortunately, today there's a complex accounting method rampant at many hospitals. They try to charge prices comparable to those for general surgery for the removal of a gallstone or kidney stone. And high tech must be allowed to stand on its own merits, not necessarily regarded as a cost center to replace another cost center. The hospital and medical community view high tech not only as a method to advance medical treatment, but also as another billing opportunity. There is a degree of unguided entrepreneurship when hospitals and physicians invest in dialysis units, magnetic resonance imaging centers, and lithotriptors.

And perhaps even the mandating or permission to use deductions for unique personal items may be controlled. As the *Wall Street Journal* reported in December 1988, the Minnesota legislature in 1987 permitted wig benefits for men and women with alopecia areata, a relatively rare disease that causes hair loss. Patients, especially women, liked the statute because wigs can cost up to $2,000.

I won't argue the wigs issue but cite it only in the context of the mounting-costs syndrome. The *New York Times* early in 1989 published an article on Medicare headlined, "Many Elderly Own Needless Health Insurance Plans." It discussed the millions of wasted dollars on extra or supplemental health insurance. The regulatory agencies, using the accountability measure, will make sure that insurers who cannot prove financial viability, meet quality-assurance standards, or satisfy peer review in cooperation with other agencies simply won't be allowed to carry on their business.

If you were to examine the seventy-seven Blue Cross plans operating today in this country, you would learn that in 1988 about sixty-six were operating with deficits reaching $3 billion in the past two years. These unprofitable plans should be obliged to prove that they understand the rating mechanisms and the cost of health care in order to live up to the accountability standards needed to sell health care to purchasers. In other words, companies buying health care insurance should not be subjected to roller-coaster rates. Those rates should be predictable and projected upon statistical performance of health care need and costs that are predicated upon the qualitative quantitative measures needed. In my opinion, the Blues are much too cozy with the hospital community. The Blues, as stated earlier in this book, view hospitals as their clients. This was clearly illustrated in Kansas City, where Blue Cross asked the hospitals for a financial "bailout" of their financial problems. Accountability would certainly change this relationship.

"By some estimates, as much as 20 percent to 30 percent of all things done by well-meaning physicians in hospitals is either inappropriate, ineffective, unnecessary and sometimes harmful," said Dr. Henry Simmons, president of the privately funded National Leadership Commission on Health Care.

The commission contends that the problems stem from uncertainty in medicine and that this could be corrected by better research and better tracking. According to Dr. Simmons, woefully little is being spent on these efforts now. Under the commission's plan, a designated percentage of a new tax will be devoted to obtaining outcome research and other related efforts. The commission was cochaired by former Iowa Governor Robert Ray and former U.S. Representative Paul Rogers of Florida. Governor Ray told reporters what many others are insisting today: There are serious problems in the quality of health care and this produces waste and in some cases even harm.

The standards of accountability so badly needed will replace much of the Band-Aid and semieffective programs being sold today to employers and insurance companies. The utilization review used in some quarters saves only a limited amount of money. And when hard-pressed in debate, there are often strong differences on who is right—the attending physician, the patient, or the reviewing agencies. Preagreed, confirmed standards of performance will, in my opinion, come into being as a joint effort of the federal government, organized medicine, and the third-party insurance carriers.

It can't fail. And everyone will benefit from it. Patients will get better care, industry and government will save money, and physicians will have the freedom to practice the high-quality medicine they want. And hospitals, too, will respond to the higher standard of accountability.

Our nation deserves nothing less than a healthy citizenry and a viable economy. As in every phase of our society, we must hold up quality as a beacon and ensure that it is always shining.

G L O S S A R Y

BLOOD PROFILE STUDIES—Multiple studies performed on blood samples usually by automated techniques pertaining to a specific area of concern, e.g., liver function profile.

CAT SCAN—An X-ray of a cross section of the body produced by a special computerized technique.

COPAYMENT—The sharing of payments, such as 10 or 20 percent or more, by the recipient of medical care.

ECHOCARDIOGRAM—A picture of the heart created on a video screen using painless sound waves, showing the size and motion of the walls and valves of the heart.

ELECTROCARDIOGRAM (EKG)—A record of the electrical activity of the heart. It may show whether the heart is normal or damaged.

EUTHANASIA—The medical term used to describe the deliberate ending of the life of an individual for reasons considered to be merciful.

FEE-FOR-SERVICE—The system for payment of medical services rendered on an itemized basis, or when the services are paid at their full charges.

FOR-PROFIT—Describes the creation of profit when services are performed in the medical delivery system. These services develop profits for the physician, the hospital, or other for-profit agencies.

HEALTH MAINTENANCE ORGANIZATIONS (HMOs)—A term coined by Paul Ellwood during the Nixon administration to describe health care organizations that were formed for the purpose of developing competition in the health care system. These organizations provide comprehensive medical benefits under a managed-care methodology.

HYPOGLYCEMIC—Having an abnormally low blood sugar level.

IATROGENIC—Term used to describe any adverse condition in a patient occurring as the result of treatment by a physician or surgeon.

INSULIN—A hormone that controls blood sugar levels and is used for the treatment of diabetes.

LITHOTRIPSY—A process for disintegrating kidney stones by using high-energy shock waves. This technique is now also being applied to the disintegration of gallstones.

MAGNETIC RESONANCE IMAGING (MRI)—A new non-X-ray technique that creates anatomic pictures by processing signals induced in body tissues by very strong magnetic forces.

MANAGED CARE—This term describes the influences introduced into the delivery and cost of health care through health care plan design patterns that monitor utilization and appropriateness of care. Attempts to negotiate the costs associated with the provision of health care standards are being related to acceptable medical protocols.

MAXIMIZERS—The billing mechanisms that providers use to bring about a maximization of financial billing. Maximizers are software methodologies used to bring about the highest possible fees in areas such as DRGs, where a higher amount of money will be received when a medical procedure is described under a different or higher relative value.

NONPROFIT—Describes a medical delivery system that is purported to operate at a level at which no profits are created. Charitable exemption requires a "gift" to the public. In other words, the value of the services to the public has to be greater than the payments received for those services, with the difference being made up by contributions, endowment income, or voluntary labor.

OCCULT BLOOD STUDIES—A method to detect hidden blood, usually in feces.

PREFERRED-PROVIDER ORGANIZATIONS (PPOs)—Providers that are preferred because of discounts provided to the medical delivery system.

PRIMARY CARE—The care rendered at the first level of entry into the medical system, usually by a family physician, internist, or pediatrician.

PROVIDERS—Physicians, dentists, and other individuals who provide services in the medical delivery system.

RELATIVE VALUE—A term used to describe the various medical complexities as weighted against a standard. Therefore, relative value scales are used to describe calculated numerical value of a procedure with consideration given to the complexities involved.

RISK SHARING—The acceptance of both the medical responsibility and the financial responsibility for the care of a patient by a medical provider or the sharing of financial risk for the care of a group of patients by groups of medical providers.

THIRD-PARTY PAYERS—Entities (insurance companies, Medicare) that pay the medical bills for people because of insurance policy, employment, or Social Security benefits.

INDEX